ANAESTHESIA
AND
CRITICAL
CARE

AN EXAM REVISION COMPANION

DATE L

MAR 2 8 2005

5 U

D1466848

Commissioning Editor: Michael Parkinson
Project Development Manager: Clive Hewat
Project Manager: Frances Affleck
Designer: Erik Bigland

PENNSYLVANIA COLLEGE OF TECHNOLOGY LIBR

6 0608 01097615 6

ANAESTHESIA
AND
CRITICAL
CARE

AN EXAM REVISION COMPANION

Chris Dodds MB BS MRCGP FRCA
Consultant Anaesthetist
James Cook University Hospital
Middlesburgh, UK

Neil Soni MBChB FANZCA FRCA FJFICM MD
Consultant in Anaesthetics and ITU
Magill Department of Anaesthetics and Intensive Care
Chelsea and Westminster Hospital
London, UK
Honorary Senior Lecturer
Imperial College Medical School
London, UK

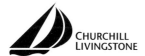
CHURCHILL
LIVINGSTONE

EDINBURGH LONDON NEW YORK OXFORD PHILADELPHIA ST LOUIS SYDNEY TORONTO
2003

LIBRARY

Pennsylvania College
of Technology

One College Avenue
Williamsport, PA 17701-5799

CHURCHILL LIVINGSTONE
An imprint of Elsevier Science Limited

JAN 1 3 2004

© 2003, Elsevier Science Limited. All rights reserved.

The right of Chris Dodds and Neil Soni to be identified as authors of this work has been asserted by them in accordance with the Copyright, Designs and Patents Act 1988.

No part of this publication may be reproduced, stored in a retrieval system, or transmitted in any form or by any means, electronic, mechanical, photocopying, recording or otherwise, without either the prior permission of the publishers or a licence permitting restricted copying in the United Kingdom issued by the Copyright Licensing Agency, 90 Tottenham Court Road, London W1T 4LP. Permissions may be sought directly from Elsevier's Health Sciences Rights Department in Philadelphia, USA: phone: (+1) 215 238 7869, fax: (+1) 215 238 2239, e-mail: healthpermissions@elsevier.com. You may also complete your request on-line via the Elsevier Science homepage (http://www.elsevier.com), by selecting 'Customer Support' and then 'Obtaining Permissions'.

First published 2003

ISBN 0443071527

British Library Cataloguing in Publication Data
A catalogue record for this book is available from the British Library

Library of Congress Cataloging in Publication Data
A catalog record for this book is available from the Library of Congress

Notice
Medical knowledge is constantly changing. Standard safety precautions must be followed, but as new research and clinical experience broaden our knowledge, changes in treatment and drug therapy may become necessary or appropriate. Readers are advised to check the most current product information provided by the manufacturer of each drug to be administered to verify the recommended dose, the method and duration of administration, and contraindications. It is the responsibility of the practitioner, relying on experience and knowledge of the patient, to determine dosages and the best treatment for each individual patient. Neither the Publisher nor the authors assumes any liability for any injury and/or damage to persons or property arising from this publication.
The Publisher

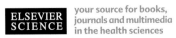

your source for books,
journals and multimedia
in the health sciences

www.elsevierhealth.com

Printed in China

Contents

Introduction

The aim of this book is to provide examination practice for candidates preparing for the final part of the FRCA examination and to assist those who help them. The book has been created by collating and updating the Continuing Medical Education sections that have appeared during the 13 years of publication of the first of the anaesthetic Continuing Education and Professional Development journals: *Current Anaesthesia and Critical Care*.

The final FRCA examination

The final FRCA examination consists of a multiple-choice question (MCQ) section, a short notes paper and two vivas, each of which has a different emphasis and requires a specific technique for successful completion. The examination uses a 'close marking' system where a pass is a score of 2, a fail is 1+ and a veto fail is 1.

The minimum score needed to pass is 2, 2, 2, 1+, but two scores of a 1+ or a single veto fail of a 1 lead to referral.[1]

The ability to pass the examination depends on both knowledge and understanding, which are tested in the written papers. The testing of judgement and clinical safety are more specifically tested in the viva examinations. However, it is important to realize that entering the oral part of the examination with a single 1+ from the written sections alters the likelihood of passing from about 70% to about 15%. This is usually a reflection of lack of knowledge and poor judgement.

This book is divided into three major sections, with a separate emphasis in each section. The first is an MCQ section, then a short notes section and finally a clinical scenario section which closely relates to the viva parts of the FRCA.

The MCQ section

The first section is a series of MCQ papers that have the same emphasis as those in the final FRCA. There are 20 questions (stems) on medical and surgical aspects related to anaesthesia and critical care, 40 questions on anaesthesia and pain management (including the basic sciences underlying these areas), 20 questions on intensive care topics and 10 questions on clinical measurement and safety. The candidates may choose to attempt a complete paper and use this to review the efficiency of their learning and recall.

There are many differing opinions on how best to answer the MCQ papers, but there are some common themes. There is certainly a minimum number of questions that have to be answered. If the pass mark is accepted as being of the

---

[1] 2+ marks are also awarded but these are only for the process of awarding medals and do not influence the outcome of a fail mark.

order of 60%, and negative marking is used, a candidate who has a 5% error will have to complete 70% of the stems to succeed. The more stems answered the better the chance of passing, until the candidate is completely guessing. Simple chance would suggest that once guessing is completely random no further marks will be scored or lost. Sadly some people guess better than others, and some will lose more marks than they score. Such 'bad guessers' should avoid gambling in this way.

There are three patterns to seek when marking the answers. The first two are seen in candidates who have a lack of knowledge. This is an insurmountable deficiency and should lead to a decision not to proceed to the examination at that time. The signs of this are of an inadequate number of questions being answered, often with visible gaps in the paper. Whole stems may be avoided, or may only have one branch answered. Another sign of borderline knowledge is where there are several attempted questions but minimal marks achieved. The final pattern is where there are isolated stems with a negative mark of −5. These are usually signs of a complete misunderstanding of a topic area or of not reading the question properly. Such a 100% error, if repeated more than once, will soon ensure failure for the candidate.

For those who are teaching the use of the MCQ, papers should be paced and used as an assessment of progress at regular intervals. The actual score should be seen to improve as the candidate's knowledge increases, but there are some hazards to using MCQs too much at this stage. Some people use MCQs to guide their learning. This is very poor technique because the areas tested are only very small fragments of the whole curriculum, and inevitably this leads to a series of knowledge gaps that will be exposed in the other parts of the examination. Another risk of too frequently repeating MCQs is that of demoralizing a candidate at a time when they need their confidence building up. Finally, there is a tendency to become focused on the minutiae of a knowledge base, whereas the majority of the examination is testing judgement and understanding. There are candidates who have encyclopaedic knowledge – and who are very good at MCQs – but who have only limited understanding and therefore rudimentary judgement.

The short notes section

The second section consists of a series of short notes questions. These are similar to those used in the short answer paper of the final FRCA (the past papers are reproduced on the RCA website: *www.rcoa.ac.uk*). This is the second of the written papers that the candidate will complete and is probably one of the most testing aspects of the examination.

The principle behind the examination is that of testing several (12) aspects of anaesthetic practice to identify the candidate's ability to balance clinical priority and judgement in a wide variety of areas. The timing for these questions is such that a descriptive essay is impossible, and short notes or headings may be all that can be used. There are several key points to remember when preparing for this paper.

All questions must be attempted. Failure to do this will lead to a fail for the paper no matter how outstanding the rest of the answers are. The order of answering the questions has been debated and there are some who recommend attempting those the candidate knows least about first, and then moving finally to the one most familiar. This is to try to avoid spending too much time on an 'expert' topic at the cost of a less well remembered one. The major disadvantage of this system is the chance of missing out a single question. Answering in sequence avoids this but does require that equal time is allotted to each question throughout.

A time of reflection before starting an individual question will allow the appropriate prioritization and clinical judgement to be displayed. Timing has to be practised both for the initial reflective organization of the answer and for the actual writing of the answer. The maximum of 15 minutes for the combined processes is very short indeed.

While there is some leeway in the marking schedule, it would be unwise to expect this to overcome more than a single area of weakness, and practice over many papers and topics is essential.

The clinical scenarios section

The viva examinations take place in London and allow the candidate to demonstrate clinical skills and experience. The clinical scenarios section is designed to be help develop good viva skills. The opportunity exists in all verbal examinations to correct initial errors and to argue the risks and benefits of a given management plan for a specific clinical dilemma. Factual knowledge and judgement are tested in the written papers but the ability to safely identify the major issues in complex cases cannot easily be tested by written papers.

Viva practice should really only start after the written papers, and should be organized with an almost military precision. While embarrassing initially, the use of a video recording of the whole process is invaluable for both parties. Setting an appropriate venue and getting several people involved are almost as important. To use only one 'examiner' makes it difficult to form questions that build on previous answers and probe areas of doubt at the same time as marking the answers and writing quotes from the answers.

Those who help prepare their colleagues for examinations have (hopefully) had very few attempts at the examination and, while enthusiastic, may not have an appropriate series of questions to use to explore clinical judgement. The series of scenarios and suggested answers are provided to use within a viva practice to explore the various, equally correct, ways of answering a single question. It is rare that a single topic fails a candidate. If there are areas of forgetfulness that appear during the practice those areas should be closed and reviewed later. Nothing but loss of confidence occurs if such areas are pursued in that session.

Introduction

Every session should end with a positive review of performance, and a suggestion of what aspects need attention before the next. Common failings, such as speaking too quietly, muttering and interjecting, are easily corrected with the use of the video. Presenting understanding rather than just knowledge is more difficult and may need to be rehearsed on many occasions. If 'examiners' are too vitriolic or abrasive to the point of making the candidate lose confidence they should be politely dropped, no matter how keen they are to help.

Good luck!

I.1   At altitude:

1   Acute mountain sickness may manifest with irritability and irrational behaviour.
2   Inspired PO_2 is calculated as $0.21 \times$ barometric pressure.
3   Initial acclimatization results in a metabolic alkalosis.
4   Acetazolamide can improve arterial PO_2.
5   Pulmonary hypertension may occur.

I.2   The following drugs, when given to patients with Parkinson's disease, have these interactions:

1   L-Dopa and halothane can cause arrhythmias.
2   L-Dopa can antagonize the anxiolytic effect of diazepam.
3   L-Dopa can cause CNS toxicity with pethidine.
4   L-Dopa can antagonize the action of metaclopamide.
5   L-Dopa acts synergistically with domperidone.

I.3   These therapeutic materials for the treatment of haemophilia have no risk of transmitting infection:

1   1-Deamino-8-D-argine vasopressin (DDAVP).
2   High-purity factor VIII concentrate.
3   Recombinant factor VIII.
4   Cryoprecipitate.
5   Intermediate-purity factor VIII concentrate.

I.4   With regard to venous air embolism, during neurosurgery:

1   It usually occurs rapidly.
2   ECG changes are a useful early sign.
3   End-tidal carbon dioxide displays are useful.
4   Central venous pressure lines placed in the right atrium reliably allow aspiration of the air.
5   A positive end-expiratory pressure of 10 cmH$_2$O helps in their prevention.

I.5   The Eaton–Lambert syndrome:

1   Occurs in 1% of patients with bronchogenic carcinoma.
2   Is associated with increased parathyroid hormone levels.
3   Causes a proximal weakness that improves with exercise.
4   Does not alter sensitivity to non-depolarizing muscle relaxants.
5   Commonly causes bulbar weakness.

I.6   **Congenital diaphragmatic hernia:**

1   Occurs in 1 in 5000 live births.
2   Has a 50% mortality within 6 hours of birth.
3   Usually presents with cyanosis, dyspnoea and cardiac dextrocardia.
4   Is rarely posterolateral (i.e. through the foramen of Bochdalek).
5   Is associated in 85% of cases with cardiovascular abnormalities.

I.7   **Cardiopulmonary bypass with hypothermia is required for the surgical correction of:**

1   Coarctation of the aorta.
2   Calcific mitral stenosis.
3   Aortic stenosis.
4   Fallot's tetralogy.
5   Constrictive pericarditis.

I.8   **Concerning secreting pituitary tumours:**

1   Visual field loss is usually unilateral.
2   Raised growth hormone production leads to excessive soft tissue enlargement.
3   Bony changes are unusual.
4   Radial artery cannulation is no more hazardous than normal.
5   The tracheal diameter is often reduced.

I.9   **Ventricular ectopic beats:**

1   Are prevented by continuous ECG monitoring.
2   May be caused by abnormalities in serum potassium concentrations.
3   Requires urgent treatment with a β-blocker.
4   Occurs uncommonly in the postoperative period.
5   Indicates underlying cardiac pathology.

I.10   **Complications of pituitary surgery include:**

1   Bleeding during a transsphenoidal approach is usually arterial secondary to the high vascularity of pituitary tumours.
2   Postoperative frontal lobe ischaemia may follow transcranial surgery.
3   Postoperative seizures are least frequent following the subfrontal approach.
4   Anosmia.
5   Diabetes insipidus.

I.11   **Vasoactive intestinal polypeptide tumours (VIPomas) may present with:**

1   Hyperglycaemia.
2   Flushing.
3   Diarrhoea.
4   Tetany from hypercalcaemia.
5   Tetany from hypomagnesaemia.

I.12   **The following signs or symptoms are typically associated with traumatic rupture of the aorta:**

1   Widened mediastinum.
2   History of penetrating chest injury.
3   Deviation of nasogastric tube to the left.
4   Elevation of the left mainstem bronchus.
5   Fracture of the upper ribs.

I.13   **The following are features of hypothyroidism:**

1   Hyponatraemia.
2   Hypokalaemia.
3   Hypoglycaemia.
4   Thrombocytopenia.
5   Anaemia.

I.14   **Acute pain crisis in sickle cell anaemia:**

1   Can be precipitated by alcohol.
2   Occurring more than three times per year significantly increases the risk of early death.
3   Should not be treated with intravenous opiates to avoid dependence.
4   Commonly involves multiple sites.
5   Is the result of reversible vasoconstriction.

I.15   **Neurofibromatosis is associated with:**

1   Paraplegia.
2   Phaeochromocytoma.
3   Renal artery stenosis.
4   Scoliosis.
5   Pulmonary fibrosis.

I.16 The following are consistent with a diagnosis of cardiac tamponade:

1 Loud first heart sound.
2 Kussmaul's respiration.
3 Basal crepitations.
4 Distended neck veins.
5 Pulsus paradoxus.

I.17 Regarding a subdural empyema:

1 It commonly produces signs of raised intracranial pressure.
2 It may be mistaken for meningitis.
3 It is treated by surgical drainage and a short course of perioperative antibiotics.
4 Neurological sequelae are rare.
5 Carries a mortality of less than 1%.

I.18 Regarding carcinoid tumours:

1 They secrete vasopressin.
2 They may produce Cushing's syndrome.
3 They are found only in the gut.
4 Carcinoid syndrome is associated with right ventricular failure.
5 Carcinoid tumour secretions are increased by raised catecholamines.

I.19 Regarding congestive cardiac failure:

1 It may occur in a patient with normal myocardial function.
2 It can result from acute fluid overload.
3 Left ventricular diastolic dysfunction alone can produce congestive cardiac failure.
4 Sudden death accounts for 40% of chronic congestive cardiac failure mortality.
5 New York Heart Association class II patients develop symptoms on less than ordinary activity.

I.20 The approximate initial incidence for neurological complications after cardiac surgery is as follows:

1 Fatal brain injury 0.5–1.0%.
2 Cognitive dysfunction 30–80%.
3 Focal brain injury (stroke) 2–5%.

4 Peripheral neuropathy 1–2%.
5 Visual field defects 25%.

I.21 **Section of the sciatic nerve at the ischial tuberosity will cause:**

1 Paralysis of the abductors of the thigh.
2 Foot drop.
3 Paralysis of the rectus femoris muscle.
4 Loss of the ankle jerk.
5 Complete loss of sensation below the knee.

I.22 **When a unit of whole blood has been stored for 14 days, the following changes are observed:**

1 The pH decreases.
2 The concentration of dextrose increases.
3 The platelet count decreases.
4 The concentration of haemoglobin within the red cells decreases.
5 The extracellular potassium concentration is likely to be less than 7 mmol l^{-1}.

I.23 **Intracranial pressure is reduced by:**

1 Ketamine.
2 Halothane.
3 Phenytoin.
4 Barbiturates.
5 Suxamethonium.

I.24 **The syndrome of supine hypotension in pregnancy:**

1 Occurs in > 50% of all pregnant patients of over 20 weeks gestation on lying supine.
2 Occurs more commonly in multiple pregnancies.
3 Is exacerbated by the administration of epidural analgesia.
4 Is avoided by the adoption of a 5° lateral tilt.
5 Is best avoided by uterine displacement to the left rather than to the right.

I.25 **Cardiac risk in patients undergoing peripheral vascular surgery:**

1 Is reliably predicted by Goldman's index.
2 Is underestimated by exercise stress tests.

3   Determines late survival as assessed by the left ventricular ejection
    fraction.
4   Should be assessed in all patients.
5   Is related to irreversible perfusion defects seen on dipyridamole–thallium
    scanning.

I.26   Difficulty in tracheal intubation should be anticipated in a patient with:

1   Pierre–Robin syndrome.
2   Sagittal synostosis.
3   Treacher–Collins syndrome.
4   Crouzon syndrome.
5   Sturge–Weber syndrome.

I.27   In the elderly patient undergoing surgery for a fracture of the femoral neck, the following are associated with a poorer outcome:

1   Increasing age.
2   Intraoperative hypotension.
3   The use of general anaesthesia.
4   Renal insufficiency.
5   Cardiac arrhythmia on the preoperative ECG.

I.28   In day-case surgery, the laryngeal mask airway:

1   Is better tolerated by patients than an endotracheal tube.
2   Is contraindicated for tonsillectomy because of the risk of aspiration.
3   Requires direct laryngoscopy for its insertion.
4   Provides a worse airway than a face mask.
5   Causes more sore throats than an endotracheal tube.

I.29   In a house fire, a young man is found with a burn injury of 30% of his body surface area. He is unconscious – barely responding to stimulation – and has acceptable ventilation and palpable peripheral pulses. The following may explain his unresponsiveness:

1   Fluid loss from the burns leading to severe hypovolaemia.
2   Hypoxia.
3   Carbon monoxide intoxication.
4   Head injury.
5   Alcohol/drug overdose.

I.30 The following statements concerning arterial baroreceptors are true:

1 They are found in the carotid sinus.
2 Their efferent fibres are carried by the glossopharyngeal nerve.
3 Stimulation of atrial baroreceptors leads to a fall in urine production via increased release of antidiuretic hormone.
4 Stimulation of carotid sinus baroreceptors results in inhibition of the vagus nerve activity.
5 Baroreceptor activity causes a rise in blood pressure.

I.31 Nitric oxide:

1 Is a naturally occurring neurotransmitter.
2 Causes smooth muscle relaxation by increasing levels of cyclic GMP.
3 Accumulates in significant levels if administered for long periods.
4 Potentiates platelet aggregation.
5 Is responsible for the action of sodium nitroprusside.

I.32 The diving reflex:

1 Is triggered by exposure of the trunk to cold water.
2 Involves the glossopharyngeal nerves in its afferent pathway.
3 Results in cerebral vasoconstriction.
4 Stimulates central chemoreceptors.
5 Is more pronounced in children than adults.

I.33 An abnormal response to suxamethonium can occur in patients with:

1 Eaton–Lambert syndrome.
2 Hepatic failure.
3 Polyarteritis nodosa.
4 Dermatomyositis.
5 Dystrophia myotonica.

I.34 Doxacurium:

1 Is a depolarizing neuromuscular relaxant.
2 Is chemically related to rocuronium.
3 Is quicker in onset than atracurium.
4 Has a similar duration of action to pancuronium.
5 Is metabolized predominantly in the liver.

I.35 The following drugs induce hepatic microsomal enzymes:

1 Enflurane.
2 Sodium valproate.
3 Isoniazid.
4 Rifampicin.
5 Phenelzine.

I.36 Regarding a jugular venous pressure waveform:

1 It reflects the pressure changes in the right atrium.
2 It is normally visible when sitting at an angle of 45°.
3 The 'a' wave occurs just before right atrial contraction.
4 Giant 'a' waves are characteristic of tricuspid regurgitation.
5 The 'c' wave is caused by closing of the pulmonary valve.

I.37 The following drugs can be used safely in a patient on long-term monoamine oxidase inhibitors:

1 Ephedrine.
2 Pethidine.
3 Ketamine.
4 Diazepam.
5 Tricyclic antidepressants.

I.38 The following reflexes produce a tachycardia:

1 Bezold–Jarisch reflex.
2 Bainbridge reflex.
3 Cushing's reflex.
4 Head's paradoxical reflex.
5 Diving reflex.

I.39 Regarding the nicotinic acetylcholine receptor:

1 It possesses four transmembrane domains.
2 Each receptor has one binding site for acetylcholine.
3 It consists of a and b subunits.
4 It is a ligand-gated ion channel receptor.
5 It is a pentamer.

I.40 **Regarding hepatitis C:**

1 It may be transmitted via blood products.
2 It is a DNA virus.
3 It rarely develops to chronic hepatitis.
4 20% recover fully from acute hepatitis C.
5 20% develop chronic active hepatitis.

I.41 **Droperidol:**

1 Is a piperazine derivative.
2 Has α-adrenergic receptor activity.
3 Produces its anti-emetic effects by acting on peripheral (D_2) dopaminergic receptors.
4 May cause extrapyramidal side effects.
5 Is predominantly excreted in the urine unchanged.

I.42 **In paediatric life support:**

1 A choking infant aged 6 months should receive abdominal thrusts if chest thrust fails to relieve airway obstruction.
2 Blind finger sweeps of the pharynx should be performed in the absence of visible airway obstruction.
3 The initial dose of adrenaline (epinephrine) in a cardiac arrest situation is $100\ \mu g\ kg^{-1}$.
4 The initial energy dose for defibrillation to treat ventricular fibrillation is $4\ J\ kg^{-1}$.
5 Intra-osseous access is only suitable for use in children under 3 years old.

I.43 **Complications of the interscalene brachial plexus block include:**

1 Pneumothorax.
2 Epidural injection.
3 Total spinal anaesthesia.
4 Intravascular injection.
5 Phrenic nerve block.

I.44 **The following drugs are of benefit in treating postherpetic neuralgia:**

1 Amitriptyline.
2 Gabapentin.
3 Lamotrigine.

4 Venlafaxine.
5 Carbamazepine.

I.45 Compared with normotensive parturients the following are raised in pre-eclampsia:

1 Fibronectin.
2 Endothelin.
3 Angiotensin II.
4 Ratio of thromboxane A_2:prostacyclin.
5 Haematocrit.

I.46 Remifentanil:

1 Is a piperidine derivative.
2 Undergoes extensive first-pass metabolism in the lung.
3 Has a prolonged duration of action in patients with suxamethonium apnoea.
4 Has a quick offset due to its large volume of distribution.
5 Does not cause muscle rigidity.

I.47 The following are associated with radial nerve injury:

1 Excessive shoulder abduction in an anaesthetized patient.
2 Loss of supination with the forearm flexed.
3 Main en griffe.
4 Loss of sensation over the lateral three and a half fingers.
5 Saturday night palsy.

I.48 Regarding folate deficiency in pregnancy:

1 It causes microcytic anaemia.
2 It is associated with neural tube defects in the fetus.
3 It is associated with cardiac defects in the fetus.
4 Diagnosis requires bone marrow biopsy.
5 Replacement is reserved for those with documented deficiency.

I.49 The following are efficacious preventative measures for the reduction of postoperative nausea and vomiting in adults:

1 Ginger powder 1 g p.o.
2 Acupressure at the P6 point.
3 Droperidol 1 mg i.v.

4 Ondansetron 1 mg i.v.
5 Dexamethasone 10 mg i.v.

I.50 **Regarding malignant hyperthermia:**

1 It is an inherited hypermetabolic disorder of smooth muscle.
2 It is triggered by non-depolarizing muscle relaxants.
3 Reconstituted dantrolene has a pH of 9 which is an irritant to veins.
4 It does not occur in children under 2 years of age.
5 It is caused by a single gene defect on chromosome 5p.

I.51 **The following are independent risk factors for pressure sore development in the critically ill:**

1 Anaemia.
2 Noradrenaline (norepinephrine) infusion for more than 60% of ICU admission.
3 Faecal incontinence for more than 3 days during ICU admission.
4 History of smoking in the past 5 years.
5 Urinary incontinence.

I.52 **Indications for the treatment of carbon monoxide poisoning with hyperbaric oxygen include:**

1 A carboxyhaemoglobin > 20% of total haemoglobin.
2 Loss of consciousness at any stage.
3 Headache.
4 Myocardial ischaemia.
5 Neurological symptoms and signs other than headache.

I.53 **The following drugs are effective treatments for post-anaesthetic shivering:**

1 Pethidine.
2 Clonidine.
3 Ketanserin.
4 Ondansetron.
5 Alfentanil.

I.54 **Regarding vecuronium:**

1 It is a bisquaternary aminosteroid.
2 It produces tachycardia via ganglion blockade.

3 It is predominantly eliminated by metabolism to deacetylated metabolites.

4 Reversal of neuromuscular blockade is unnecessary if more than 40 minutes have passed since the last bolus of vecuronium.

5 A train-of-four ratio greater than 0.7 indicates adequate enough recovery from neuromuscular block to prevent passive regurgitation and aspiration.

I.55   **The following should be avoided in porphyria:**

1 Etomidate.

2 Hartmann's solution.

3 Halothane.

4 Indomethacin.

5 Alfentanil.

I.56   **Compared to bupivacaine, ropivacaine:**

1 Has a higher pK_a.

2 Is more lipid soluble.

3 Blocks type C nerve fibres faster.

4 Blocks type A nerve fibres more slowly.

5 Is less cardiotoxic.

I.57   **Suggested causes of neurological dysfunction seen after cardiopulmonary bypass include:**

1 Gaseous macroemboli.

2 Lipid microemboli.

3 Nitrous oxide.

4 Glutamate toxicity.

5 Cerebral hypoperfusion.

I.58   **As an in-vivo buffer, THAM (tris-hydroxymethyl-aminomethane) has the following advantages over sodium bicarbonate:**

1 Less sodium load.

2 It does not increase $PaCO_2$.

3 Less irritation to peripheral veins.

4 It does not cross the blood–brain barrier.

5 Less respiratory depression.

I.59 Following inadvertent dural puncture:

1 A prophylactic blood patch is contraindicated.
2 A blood patch within 24 hours is contraindicated.
3 An epidural saline infusion will decrease the likelihood that a blood patch will be required subsequently.
4 If headache develops, a blood patch would be expected to confer a 50% chance of persistent relief.
5 If a blood patch is performed, subsequent epidural analgesia is likely to be ineffective.

I.60 Cricoid pressure:

1 Is less reliably sustained using the non-dominant hand.
2 May prevent mask ventilation.
3 Can interfere with laryngoscopy if incorrectly applied.
4 Can be effectively sustained for 20 minutes in emergency situations.
5 Is of proven benefit.

I.61 When monitoring a ventilated 6-month-old child:

1 The sampling rate of the capnograph should be very low.
2 A transcutaneous CO_2 electrode will underestimate the $PaCO_2$.
3 Non-invasive blood pressure measurement will be inaccurate.
4 The shape of the S–T component of the QRS complex is rarely clinically important.
5 Pulse oximetry gives a good estimate of the true oxyhaemoglobin saturation.

I.62 The most important influences on intensive care mortality include:

1 Mechanical ventilation.
2 Emergency surgery.
3 Age.
4 Malignancy.
5 Timing of therapy.

I.63 Regarding spinal injuries:

1 Spinal shock is caused by parasympathetic paralysis.
2 Shock may be due to haemorrhage or impaired cardiac function.
3 Suxamethonium may be used in the first 24 hours post injury.

4   All cervical spinal injuries lead to limited expiratory function.

5   Tracheal suctioning may precipitate bradycardia.

I.64   **The following are true of phosphate homeostasis:**

1   Phosphate is the most abundant intracellular anion.

2   Standard laboratory tests measure total serum phosphate.

3   Serum phosphate levels give an accurate indication of total body phosphate stores.

4   Patients with chronic obstructive pulmonary disease have a higher incidence of hypophosphataemia than those without respiratory disease.

5   Rapid correction of hypophosphataemia has been associated with renal failure.

I.65   **Low serum phosphate may result from treatment with:**

1   Sodium citrate.

2   Dopamine.

3   Acetazolamide.

4   Theophylline.

5   Paracetamol.

I.66   **Perfluorocarbons:**

1   If instilled into lungs are not absorbed systemically.

2   Have been used successfully as substitutes for blood transfusion.

3   Are able to transport oxygen but not carbon dioxide.

4   During liquid ventilation do not interfere with chest X-ray interpretation.

5   Their high density is thought to be in part responsible for their beneficial actions in liquid ventilation.

I.67   **Regarding partial liquid ventilation in patients with adult respiratory distress syndrome (ARDS):**

1   It requires a specialized ventilator.

2   It involves the instillation of perfluorocarbon equivalent to the estimated residual volume.

3   It improves both oxygenation and compliance.

4   In contrast to conventional (gas) ventilation, the lung is ventilated in a more uniform manner.

5   The beneficial effects of partial liquid ventilation on oxygenation have been shown to be due to redistribution of pulmonary blood flow.

I.68 **Regarding renal replacement therapy in a patient with acute renal failure complicating acute liver failure:**

1 Cerebral oedema is an indication to start therapy.
2 Haemodialysis is the treatment of choice.
3 Anticoagulation of the circuit is rarely required.
4 Bicarbonate buffering solutions should be used.
5 Epoprostenol may be useful.

I.69 **The following are recognized causes of disseminated intravascular coagulation (DIC):**

1 Viraemia.
2 Heatstroke.
3 Following snake-bite.
4 Cirrhosis.
5 Amniotic fluid embolism.

I.70 **In the diagnosis of a blast injury:**

1 Eardrum perforation is present in 85% of cases.
2 Laryngeal petechiae are often insignificant.
3 Pulmonary blast injury may be asymptomatic for some hours.
4 An association with other trauma is uncommon.
5 Asymptomatic patients from within the blast area may be sent home.

I.71 **Regarding paraquat:**

1 It is usually fatal if more than 15 ml is ingested.
2 Gut absorption is initially high.
3 Severe diarrhoea is common and may complicate fluid balance.
4 High concentrations of oxygen are required in the early management phase.
5 Pulmonary fibrosis is the usual cause of death.

I.72 **In the management of burns:**

1 Mortality has improved by 50% for young patients.
2 Central venous pressure and urine output provide appropriate guides to fluid therapy.
3 Evaporative losses are of the order of 2 ml kg^{-1} h^{-1}.

4   A hoarse voice indicates significant airway injury.
5   Invasive monitoring lines should be placed directly through burned areas to reduce the pain of insertion.

I.73   *Pneumocystis carinii* pneumonia:

1   Is the commonest infection in HIV-positive patients.
2   Carries a poor prognosis if ventilatory support is required.
3   Is not associated with an increased risk of pneumothorax.
4   Should be treated with steroids at an early stage.
5   Pentamidine is the first-line antibiotic in most patients.

I.74   Gastric secretions are increased by:

1   Secretin.
2   Vagal stimulation.
3   Sympathetic stimulation.
4   Gastrin secretion.
5   Acidic stomach contents.

I.75   The following drugs should be administered in reduced dosage in severe renal failure:

1   Amiodarone.
2   Cefuroxime.
3   Digoxin.
4   Gentamicin.
5   Benzylpenicillin.

I.76   In the treatment of acute head injury:

1   Mannitol has been proven to be more effective than placebo.
2   Barbiturates reduce cerebral blood flow to non-injured brain.
3   Prophylactic hyperventilation has a beneficial effect.
4   Hypothermia is associated with increased medical complications.
5   Much of the secondary injury occurs after admission to hospital.

I.77   The addition of positive end-expiratory pressure during mechanical ventilation:

1   Increases the risk of a pneumothorax.
2   Reduces extravascular lung water (EVLW).

3   Generally improves arterial oxygenation.
4   Depresses cardiac output mainly by increasing right ventricular afterload.
5   Increases renal sodium loss.

I.78   Considering high-frequency jet ventilation (HFJV):

1   Ventilator minute volume varies with frequency.
2   An increase in inspiratory time increases lung volume.
3   It works best at frequencies between 180 and 240 breaths min^{-1}.
4   A decrease in driving pressure causes an increase in the arterial PCO_2.
5   Pulmonary ventilation is always the same as the minute volume determined by the ventilator controls.

I.79   In the treatment of adult respiratory distress syndrome (ARDS) the following are likely to be of benefit:

1   High-dose steroids.
2   Prophylactic antibiotics.
3   Concentrations of oxygen of 80–100%.
4   Fluid replacement with crystalloids only.
5   The administration of a pulmonary vasodilator.

I.80   Cardiac tamponade:

1   May occur with a penetrating injury to the abdomen.
2   May occur post cardiac surgery.
3   Classically causes a triad of hypotension, raised central venous pressure and quiet heart sounds.
4   Is a cause of non-VF/VT cardiac arrest.
5   Is definitively treated by needle pericardiocentesis.

I.81   Concerning these physical laws:

1   Henry's law states that the amount of gas dissolved is proportional to the partial pressure of the gas.
2   Charles' law states that the volume of gas is inversely proportional to the change in temperature.
3   A change in pressure or volume of a gas that occurs without an energy change is adiabatic.
4   Graham's law states that the rate of diffusion of a gas is proportional to the square of the molecular weight.
5   Fick's law states that the rate of diffusion across a membrane is proportional to the thickness of that membrane.

I.82 The following are SI units:

1 The gram.
2 The newton.
3 The joule.
4 The second.
5 Degrees celsius.

I.83 The following are true of nitrous oxide:

1 It is a non-halogenated hydrocarbon.
2 Is of benefit as it is rarely associated with nausea and vomiting.
3 It exhibits the Poynting effect when stored in its pure form.
4 It is less dense than air.
5 It has a critical pressure of 36.5 bar.

I.84 In a normal person breathing air:

1 Arterial blood contains approximately 20 ml of dissolved oxygen per 100 ml.
2 Each gram of haemoglobin carries 1.39 ml of oxygen.
3 The oxyhaemoglobin dissociation curve shifts to the left in the pulmonary capillaries.
4 Arterial blood contains around 2.5 ml of dissolved carbon dioxide per 100 ml.
5 The majority of carbon dioxide in venous blood is carried as carbamino compounds.

I.85 The following are parametric statistical tests:

1 Chi-square test.
2 Fisher's exact test.
3 Student's t-test.
4 Paired t-test.
5 Wilcoxon signed rank test.

I.86 The following are appropriate methods of measuring volatile agents in a mixture of gases:

1 Fuel cell.
2 Piezo-electric resonance.
3 Raman spectrometry.
4 Infrared spectroscopy.
5 Mass spectrometry.

I.87 Regarding turbulent flow of gases in a breathing system:

1 Flow is directly proportional to pressure.
2 Decreasing the diameter of the tubing by half will decrease the flow by a factor of 16.
3 The gas viscosity is more important in determining flow than its density.
4 Turbulent flow will occur if the Reynolds number is 2000 or more.
5 It occurs at higher flow rates as the gases are warmed.

I.88 100 mmHg pressure is approximately equal to:

1 13.3 kPa.
2 147 cmH_2O.
3 1 bar.
4 14.5 psi.
5 100 torr.

I.89 Regarding brainstem auditory evoked potentials (BAEPs):

1 They measure the electrical potentials produced by the brainstem and cortex in response to auditory stimuli.
2 Short-latency (<10 ms) responses assess only auditory cortex function.
3 Transient BAEPs consist of a series of positive and negative waves.
4 Awareness can occur if anaesthesia is maintained using drugs that preserve middle-latency auditory-evoked potentials (MLAEPs).
5 Propofol suppresses the MLAEPs.

I.90 Regarding the measurement of gastric intramucosal PCO_2:

1 When employing conventional tonometry, a buffered tonometer solution is preferred.
2 Saline gives greater precision than air as the tonometer medium.
3 A pHi less than 7.32 is a very specific indicator of gastrointestinal malperfusion.
4 A pHi less than 7.32 is a very sensitive indicator of mortality in critically ill patients.
5 Experimentally, metabolic decompensation occurs at a blood flow reduction of 60%.

I.1   At altitude:

1 True   2 False   3 False   4 True   5 True

When ascending to altitudes of 2000 m and above, symptoms will be experienced by the unacclimatized due to a decrease in inspired PO_2. This is calculated as 0.21 (barometric pressure – saturated vapour pressure). Initially there may be an awareness of increased breathlessness on exertion, accompanied by headache, nausea, anorexia and insomnia. At 5000 m, dyspnoea will be experienced at rest, along with dizziness and loss of memory. Periodic apnoeas during sleep become common. Acute mountain sickness may be life threatening when pulmonary and/or cerebral oedema develops, normally at altitudes above 3000 m. The aetiology of pulmonary oedema is not clearly understood but pulmonary hypertension secondary to hypoxic pulmonary vasoconstriction is described. Cerebral oedema may manifest as ataxia or irrational behaviour, progressing to coma. Treatment involves oxygen therapy and descent to lower altitude. Acetazolamide may be used to assist acclimatization.

I.2   The following drugs, when given to patients with Parkinson's disease, have these interactions:

1 True   2 True   3 False   4 True   5 False

I.3   These therapeutic materials for the treatment of haemophilia have no risk of transmitting infection:

1 True   2 False   3 True   4 False   5 False

I.4   With regard to venous air embolism, during neurosurgery:

1 False   2 False   3 True   4 False   5 True

I.5   The Eaton–Lambert syndrome:

1 True   2 True   3 True   4 False   5 False

I.6   Congenital diaphragmatic hernia:

1 True   2 True   3 True   4 False   5 False

I.7 Cardiopulmonary bypass with hypothermia is required for the surgical correction of:

| 1 False | 2 True | 3 True | 4 True | 5 False |

Cardiopulmonary bypass with hypothermia to reduce metabolic rate is required for open heart procedures and coronary artery bypass grafting.

Coarctation repair involves either resection of the affected segment with end-to-end anastomosis or reconstruction with a subclavian flap or Dacron patch. It is normally undertaken under deep hypothermia and aortic cross-clamping, although left-sided bypass has been used. Closed or open valvotomy is suitable for patients with mobile, non-calcified non-regurgitant mitral valves and will produce good results for 10 years or more. Mitral valve replacement is indicated for calcified valves.

I.8 Concerning secreting pituitary tumours:

| 1 False | 2 True | 3 False | 4 False | 5 True |

I.9 Ventricular ectopic beats:

1 False
2 True
3 False. Treatment is only required if the beats are either very frequent or are associated a fall in cardiac output.
4 False
5 False. They occur commonly in normal individuals.

I.10 Complications of pituitary surgery include:

| 1 True | 2 True | 3 False | 4 False | 5 False |

I.11 Vasoactive intestinal polypeptide tumours (VIPomas) may present with:

| 1 True | 2 True | 3 True | 4 True | 5 True |

I.12 The following signs or symptoms are typically associated with traumatic rupture of the aorta:

1 True
2 False. The mechanism is usually sudden deceleration – road traffic accident or a fall.

3 False. Deviation of the nasogastric tube is to the right.
4 False. Depression of the left mainstem bronchus.
5 True

I.13 The following are features of hypothyroidism:

1 True 2 False 3 True 4 False 5 True

I.14 Acute pain crisis in sickle cell anaemia:

1 True 2 True 3 False 4 True 5 False

I.15 Neurofibromatosis is associated with:

1 True 2 True 3 True 4 True 5 True

Neurofibromatosis (von Recklinghausen's disease) is characterized by peripheral and central neurofibromas. Spinal cord tumours may result in paraplegia. One percent of patients develop a phaeochromocytoma.

I.16 The following are consistent with a diagnosis of cardiac tamponade:

1 False 2 False 3 False 4 True 5 True

The heart sounds are usually muffled although relative accentuation of the pulmonary component of S2 may be present. The lungs are clear to auscultation, and the neck veins are distended. Kussmaul's sign (inspiratory distension of neck veins) may be present if there is coexisting epicardial constriction. Pulsus paradoxus (inspiratory decrease in systolic pressure) is usually detectable by palpation.

I.17 Regarding a subdural empyema:

1 True 2 True 3 False 4 False 5 False

Antibiotics should be continued for 3–6 weeks. Neurological sequelae are common. Mortality is in excess of 10%.

I.18 Regarding carcinoid tumours:

1 False 2 False 3 False 4 True 5 True

Seventy-five percent of carcinoid tumours arise in the gut, with those in the foregut producing more serotonin (5-HT) than the more common ones that arise from the midgut (most usually the appendix). The 5-HT levels can be so high as to lead to pulmonary hypertension and thus to right heart failure.

I.19	Regarding congestive cardiac failure:

1 True	2 True	3 True	4 True	5 False

New York Heart Association (NYHA) class II patients develop symptoms on slight, mild, limited activity; it is class III patients who have marked limitation of activity and are only comfortable at rest.

I.20	The approximate initial incidence for neurological complications after cardiac surgery is as follows:

1 False	2 True	3 True	4 False	5 True

I.21	Section of the sciatic nerve at the ischial tuberosity will cause:

1 False	2 True	3 False	4 True	5 False

The sciatic nerve is one of two terminal branches of the sacral plexus and is derived from the anterior primary rami of L4,5 S1–3 roots. It is the largest peripheral nerve in the body. The sciatic nerve leaves the pelvis through the greater sciatic foramen and runs roughly halfway between the ischial tuberosity and the greater trochanter to enter the thigh, where it descends vertically down the midline of the back of the leg until the popliteal fossa is reached. At this point it divides into the common peroneal nerve and the tibial nerve. The sciatic nerve supplies the hamstrings and the muscles of the lower leg. It mediates sensation from the lateral side of the calf and most of the foot apart from the medial edge, which is supplied by the femoral nerve.

I.22	When a unit of whole blood has been stored for 14 days, the following changes are observed:

1 True	2 False	3 True	4 True	5 False

Whole blood is not widely available, rather the emphasis has been on blood component therapy to meet specific transfusion requirements. However, it does have the advantage of providing red blood cells and plasma proteins with a single donor exposure. Most clotting factors are relatively stable in storage, but factors V and VIII will fall to 10–20% over the first 2 weeks. There will be few functional platelets in stored blood. Approximately 450 ml of donated blood are mixed with 63 ml of citrate phosphate dextrose anticoagulant resulting in a haematocrit of 35–45%. Adenine is added to help maintain ATP levels and improve red cell survival. A pack will last 35 days when stored at $4°C \pm 2°C$. Ongoing red cell metabolism consumes dextrose, and produces hydrogen ions and potassium. Nearing the end of its shelf-life blood may have a potassium concentration of 25–30 mmol l^{-1}.

I.23 Intracranial pressure is reduced by:

1 False   2 False   3 False   4 True   5 False

The cranium is essentially a closed container and intracranial pressure (ICP) is therefore directly related to the volume of its contents, namely tissue, blood and water. The agents listed affect the ICP through their effect on cerebral blood flow. Increasing cerebral blood flow will increase ICP and reducing cerebral blood flow will reduce ICP. Phenytoin has no direct effect and indeed may reduce cerebral blood flow if its administration results in the cessation of seizure activity. The evidence surrounding suxamethonium is controversial and it has been argued that any increase in ICP seen after suxamethonium is the result of inadequate anaesthesia rather than muscle fasciculations.

I.24 The syndrome of supine hypotension in pregnancy:

1 False. The reported incidence is 11%.
2 True
3 True. The sympathetic blockade may interfere with the baroreceptor-regulated compensation if the block is high.
4 False. At least 15–20° of tilt is recommended.
5 True

I.25 Cardiac risk in patients undergoing peripheral vascular surgery:

1 False. Goldman's index underestimates cardiac events in patients at low risk.
2 True. Vascular patients may not be capable of exercising enough, but inotrope-induced stress testing is helpful.
3 True. Ejection fractions below 50% predict an increased risk of death, and if below 30% indicate a threefold increase in mortality at 12 weeks.
4 True
5 False. The risk is related to reversible defects that indicate areas of hypoperfusion.

I.26 Difficulty in tracheal intubation should be anticipated in a patient with:

1 True
2 False
3 True
4 True. Not always, but the size of the mandible may be underestimated because of maxillary hypoplasia.
5 False.

I.27 In the elderly patient undergoing surgery for a fracture of the femoral neck, the following are associated with a poorer outcome:

1 True   2 False   3 False   4 True   5 True

Outcome for surgery for a hip fracture is determined by the general status of the patient on admission. Increasing age, ischaemic heart disease, cardiac failure, preoperative arrhythmias on ECG, high ASA status (3 and 4), dementia and possibly male gender are all associated with increased mortality. The evidence one way or another for general or regional anaesthesia is still not strong but suggests that regional may be safer. Postoperatively pneumonia, renal failure and cerebrovascular accidents significantly increase mortality.

I.28 In day-case surgery, the laryngeal mask airway:

1 True   2 False   3 False   4 False   5 False

The laryngeal mask airway is better tolerated than an endotracheal tube at lower anaesthetic depth and with fewer sore throats. It is easily inserted and provides a more secure and reliable airway than a face mask.

I.29 In a house fire, a young man is found with a burn injury of 30% of his body surface area. He is unconscious – barely responding to stimulation – and has acceptable ventilation and palpable peripheral pulses. The following may explain his unresponsiveness:

1 False   2 True   3 True   4 True   5 True

I.30 The following statements concerning arterial baroreceptors are true:

1 True   2 False   3 False   4 False   5 False

Baroreceptors are stretch receptors. They are found in the walls of arteries, veins and the heart chambers. The question concerns only the arterial receptors and so, while stimulation of atrial baroreceptors does indeed increase ADH secretion, the answer is false. Arterial baroreceptors are found in the carotid sinus and the aortic arch. The two different sites send their afferent signals to the medulla by different nerves. The carotid receptors send their impulses via the carotid sinus nerve, which is a branch of the glossopharyngeal nerve, while the vagus carries impulses from the aortic arch receptors. Stimulation of these baroreceptors results in inhibition of the vasomotor centre and excitation of the cardio-inhibitory centre. This results in vasodilatation due to reduced sympathetic output and bradycardia due to increased vagal activity.

I.31 Nitric oxide:

1 True   2 True   3 False   4 False   5 True

Nitric oxide is an endogenous mediator of vascular dilatation, neurotransmission, immune defence and inhibition of platelet adhesion. In vascular smooth muscle it activates guanylyl cyclase, generating cyclic GMP. This decreases the amount of intracellular calcium ion available for smooth muscle contraction. Sodium nitroprusside and glyceryl trinitrate release intracellular nitric oxide, resulting in their vasodilatory actions. Activation of platelet guanylyl cyclase decreases platelet intracellular calcium, resulting in a decrease in platelet adhesiveness. Nitric oxide has a half-life of 3–50 seconds, being rapidly inactivated by haemoglobin. Thus its effects are limited to its site of release, preventing accumulation from occurring.

I.32 The diving reflex:

1 False   2 False   3 False   4 False   5 True

The diving reflex is triggered by the exposure of the face to cold water. Stimulation of the trigeminal nerves produces peripheral vasoconstriction and a vagally mediated bradycardia. The cerebral and cardiac circulations are preserved. Chemoreceptor and baroreceptor function is overridden. The reflex is more pronounced in children than in adults.

I.33 An abnormal response to suxamethonium can occur in patients with:

1 True   2 True   3 True   4 True   5 True

Patients with Eaton–Lambert syndrome show exaggerated responses to depolarizing and non-depolarizing relaxants. Impaired liver function can result in low levels of plasma cholinesterase. Polyarteritis nodosa and dermatomyositis may cause liver dysfunction. Prolonged muscle contraction can result in patients with dystrophia myotonica if they are given suxamethonium.

I.34	Doxacurium:

1 False	2 False	3 False	4 True	5 False

Doxacurium is a non-depolarizing relaxant belonging to the benzylquinolinium group of drugs. Other drugs in this group include atracurium and mivacurium. Rocuronium is an aminosteroid. Doxacurium has a similar duration of action to pancuronium but is slightly slower in onset. It is metabolized in the plasma.

I.35	The following drugs induce hepatic microsomal enzymes:

1 True	2 False	3 False	4 True	5 False

Valproate, isoniazid and phenelzine (a monoamine oxidase inhibitor) inhibit hepatic microsomal enzymes.

I.36	Regarding a jugular venous pressure waveform:

1 True	2 True	3 False	4 False	5 False

The jugulous venous pressure is a delayed refection of the pressure changes in the right atrium. Tricuspid regurgitation causes giant 'cv' waves. The 'c' wave is caused by bulging of the tricuspid valve into the right atrium during ventricular contraction.

I.37	The following drugs can be used safely in a patient on long-term monoamine oxidase inhibitors:

1 False	2 False	3 False	4 True	5 False

I.38	The following reflexes produce a tachycardia:

1 False	2 True	3 False	4 False	5 False

The Bezold–Jarisch reflex causes bradycardia and hypotension following rapid infusion of fluid. Cushing's reflex is bradycardia and hypertension with an increase in intracranial pressure. Head's paradoxical reflex is a lung reflex seen in rabbits. The diving reflex causes a bradycardia following immersion of the face in water.

I.39   Regarding the nicotinic acetylcholine receptor:

1 True   2 False   3 True   4 True   5 True

Each receptor has two binding sites for acetylcholine.

I.40   Regarding hepatitis C:

1 True   2 False   3 False   4 True   5 True

Hepatitis C is an RNA virus. Fifty to eighty percent of patients develop chronic hepatitis from acute hepatitis C infection.

I.41   Droperidol:

1 False   2 True   3 False   4 True   5 False

Droperidol is a butyrophenone derivative. Droperidol can produce hypotension in the presence of hypovolaemia. Droperidol's anti-emetic effects are brought about through central action on the chemoreceptor trigger zone (CTZ). Droperidol is extensively metabolized by the liver to leave only 1% excreted unchanged.

I.42   In paediatric life support:

1 False   2 False   3 False   4 False   5 False

Abdominal thrusts should not be used in children aged under 1 year. Blind finger sweeps are not recommended. Adrenaline (epinephrine) dosage is 10 μg kg^{-1} initially. 2 J kg^{-1} should be used initially for defibrillation to treat ventricular fibrillation. Intra-osseous access can be used in all children and even in adults, although gaining access is more difficult.

I.43   Complications of the interscalene brachial plexus block include:

1 False   2 True   3 True   4 True   5   True

I.44   The following drugs are of benefit in treating postherpetic neuralgia:

1 True   2 True   3 True   4 True   5 True

I.45 Compared with normotensive parturients, the following are raised in pre-eclampsia:

1 True   2 True   3 False   4 True   5 True

Fibronectin is a marker of endothelial damage and endothelin is a potent vasoconstrictor. Endothelial damage and vasoconstriction are prominent features of pre-eclampsia. Levels of angiotensin II are higher in the pregnant than non-pregnant state but in pre-eclampsia, however, the levels are lower. Thromboxane A_2 and prostacyclin have opposing effects on the vascular system. Thromboxane causes vasoconstriction and platelet aggregation. Relative levels of thromboxane are greater in pre-eclampsia. Plasma volume depletion leads to haemoconcentration.

(Norris MC. *Handbook of Obstetric Anaesthesia*. Lippincott Williams & Wilkins, 2000: 104–119.)

I.46 Remifentanil:

1 True   2 False   3 False   4 False   5 False

Remifentanil is a piperidine derivative that is metabolized by non-specific esterases in blood and other tissues, although the lung is not thought to play a large part in its degradation. Its breakdown is unaltered by plasma cholinesterase levels. Remifentanil has a small volume of distribution, its rapid offset being due to redistribution within this volume and rapid metabolism. In common with all opioids, remifentanil may cause muscle rigidity in high doses.

(Glass PSA, Tong JG, Howell S. A review of the pharmacokinetics and pharmacodynamics of remifentanil. *Anesth Analg* 1999; 89: S7–14.)

I.47 The following are associated with radial nerve injury:

1 False   2 False   3 False   4 False   5 True

The radial nerve is classically damaged by pressure in the axilla by a crutch or by an alcohol-induced sleep with an arm hanging over the back of a chair – the Saturday night palsy. If the main trunk is damaged, supination of the *extended* forearm is lost. When flexed, however, the biceps are able to perform this movement. Only a small patch of sensation is lost between the thumb and forefinger. Main en griffe or claw hand is a feature of ulnar nerve injuries.

I.48 Regarding folate deficiency in pregnancy:

1 False   2 True   3 False   4 False   5 False

Folate deficiency is the largest cause of macrocytic anaemia in pregnancy. Severe deficiency has been associated with neural tube defects and cleft palates but not cardiac defects. It is diagnosed on a peripheral blood smear. Folate supplementation is routinely given to virtually all pregnant women.

I.49 The following are efficacious preventative measures for the reduction of postoperative nausea and vomiting in adults:

1 False   2 True   3 True   4 True   5 True

I.50 Regarding malignant hyperthermia:

1 False   2 False   3 True   4 False   5 False

I.51 The following are independent risk factors for pressure sore development in the critically ill:

1 True   2 True   3 True   4 False   5 False

I.52 Indications for the treatment of carbon monoxide poisoning with hyperbaric oxygen include:

1 True   2 True   3 False   4 True   5 True

I.53 The following drugs are effective treatments for post-anaesthetic shivering:

1 True   2 True   3 True   4 True   5 True

I.54 Regarding vecuronium:

1 False   2 False   3 False   4 False   5 False

I.55 The following should be avoided in porphyria:

1 True   2 False   3 False   4 False   5 False

I.56 Compared to bupivacaine, ropivacaine:

1 False   2 False   3 False   4 True   5 True

I.57 Suggested causes of neurological dysfunction seen after cardiopulmonary bypass include:

1 True   2 True   3 False   4 True   5 True

I.58 As an in-vivo buffer, THAM (tris-hydroxymethyl-aminomethane) has the following advantages over sodium bicarbonate:

1 True   2 True   3 False   4 False   5 False

I.59 Following inadvertent dural puncture:

1 False   2 False   3 False   4 False   5 False

I.60 Cricoid pressure:

1 True   2 True   3 True   4 False   5 False

I.61 When monitoring a ventilated 6-month-old child:

1 False. If the sampling is too slow the profile displayed will be inaccurate and misleading.
2 False. Transcutaneous measurements usually overestimate the $PaCO_2$.
3 False. The readings will be accurate provided an appropriate cuff size is used.
4 True. Rate and rhythm are more informative, especially as precise placement of electrodes on children is more difficult and clear interpretation therefore less accurate.
5 True. Fetal haemoglobin has little effect on the accuracy.

I.62 The most important influences on intensive care mortality include:

1 False   2 False   3 True   4 False   5 True

Emergency surgery and mechanical ventilation are associated with more severe physiological disturbance but are not by themselves prime determinants of survival, unlike the timing of therapy and age. Elderly patients do have a higher mortality, as have those who have been ill for some time.

I.63	Regarding spinal injuries:
	1 False 2 True 3 True 4 True 5 True

High lesions cause sympathetic paralysis.

I.64	The following are true of phosphate homeostasis:
	1 True 2 False 3 False 4 True 5 True

I.65	Low serum phosphate may result from treatment with:
	1 False 2 True 3 True 4 True 5 False

I.66	Perfluorocarbons:
	1 False 2 True 3 False 4 False 5 True

I.67	Regarding partial liquid ventilation in patients with acute respiratory distress syndrome (ARDS):
	1 False 2 False 3 True 4 True 5 False

I.68	Regarding renal replacement therapy in a patient with acute renal failure complicating acute liver failure:
	1 True 2 False 3 False 4 True 5 True

I.69	The following are recognized causes of disseminated intravascular coagulation (DIC):
	1 True 2 True 3 True 4 True 5 True

I.70	In the diagnosis of a blast injury:
1 True	2 False	3 True	4 False	5 False

Blast injury occurs when an organism is exposed to the effects of a strong explosion or a shock wave. Either the initial intensely high-pressure change or the displaced volume of air can cause tissue disruption. The commonest injury is a perforated eardrum and this is an indication of the severity of the injury and a marker of possible pulmonary effects. Laryngeal petechiae are always significant signs of a severe pulmonary/airway injury, and this injury may not present for some hours. However, inspection of the larynx may be hazardous. The nearer the patient to the blast area, the more likely they are to have associated injuries, especially in an underwater explosion. Certainly those near an explosion should be kept under close observation.

(Saissy JM. Blast injury. *Curr Anaesth Crit Care* 1998; 9: 58–65.)

I.71	Regarding paraquat:
1 True	2 False	3 True	4 False	5 True

I.72	In the management of burns:
1 True	2 False	3 True	4 True	5 False

The calculation of age minus the percentage of third-degree burn to equate to mortality is still accurate above the age of 65 years, but the mortality in younger patients has been reduced by half.

I.73	*Pneumocystis carinii* pneumonia:
1 True	2 True	3 False	4 True	5 False

I.74	Gastric secretions are increased by:
1 False	2 True	3 False	4 True	5 False

I.75	The following drugs should be administered in reduced dosage in severe renal failure:
1 False	2 True	3 True	4 True	5 True

I.76	In the treatment of acute head injury:

| 1 False | 2 True | 3 False | 4 True | 5 False |

I.77	The addition of positive end-expiratory pressure during mechanical ventilation:

| 1 True | 2 False | 3 True | 4 False | 5 False |

Increasing airway pressure increases the risk of barotrauma. The EVLW is unchanged or even rises slightly, but is redistributed away from the alveolae. Arterial oxygenation is improved but because of the potential fall in cardiac output oxygen delivery may still fall. Remember oxygen flux is O_2 content × cardiac output. The prime cause for the fall in cardiac output is a reduction in venous return. Only where there is severe right heart failure will the afterload become a significant factor. Sodium is retained due to increased levels of aldosterone.

I.78	Considering high-frequency jet ventilation (HFJV):

| 1 False | 2 True | 3 False | 4 True | 5 False |

The minute volume increases with the driving pressure and inspiratory time. Frequency changes have no effect because the total inspiratory time each minute remains the same. The lung volume is greater with longer inspiratory times because the expiratory time is reduced. The end-expiratory pressure that develops increases lung volume according to thoracic compliance. HFJV has an optimal frequency of 60–120 breaths min^{-1}. Decreasing driving pressure reduces minute ventilation, leading to a rise in CO_2.

I.79	In the treatment of adult respiratory distress syndrome (ARDS) the following are likely to be of benefit:

| 1 False | 2 True | 3 False | 4 False | 5 True |

Steroids have no proven benefit, while prophylactic antibiotics may be helpful because sepsis increases mortality. High inspired oxygen concentrations may be necessary but are not directly beneficial.

I.80	Cardiac tamponade:

| 1 True | 2 True | 3 True | 4 True | 5 False |

Definitive treatment depends upon the cause of the tamponade.

I.81 Concerning these physical laws:

1 True   2 False   3 True   4 False   5 False

I.82 The following are base SI units:

1 False   2 False   3 False   4 True   5 False

There are seven base SI units: metre, second, kilogram, ampere, kelvin, candela and mole. From these base units many other derived units such as the newton and the joule may be obtained.

I.83 The following are true of nitrous oxide:

1 False   2 False   3 False   4 False   5 False

Nitrous oxide is an inorganic gas. It causes nausea and vomiting in up to 15% of patients. The Poynting effect, also known as the overpressure effect, refers to the dissolution of gaseous oxygen when it is bubbled through liquid N_2O, and the ensuing vaporization of the liquid N_2O to form a gaseous O_2/N_2O mixture. Nitrous oxide has a specific gravity of 1.53 and is therefore more dense than air. It has a critical pressure of 71.7 atmospheres, meaning that this is the pressure required to liquefy gaseous N_2O when it is at its critical temperature (36.5 °C).

I.84 In a normal person breathing air:

1 False   2 False   3 True   4 True   5 False

Arterial blood normally carries 20 ml of oxygen per 100 ml, only 0.3 ml of which is in solution. Haemoglobin can theoretically carry 1.39 ml of oxygen per gram but *in vivo*, because of impurities, e.g. methaemoglobin, the value is closer to 1.34 ml g^{-1}. As blood passes through the pulmonary capillary carbon dioxide diffuses from it, reducing the carbonic acid content and hydrogen ion content. This causes a left shift in the oxyhaemoglobin dissociation curve. The majority of carbon dioxide is carried as bicarbonate. Venous blood carries only 3.5 ml as carbamino compounds from a total of 54 ml.

I.85 The following are parametric statistical tests:

1 False   2 False   3 True   4 True   5 False

I.86 The following are appropriate methods of measuring volatile agents in a mixture of gases:

1 False 2 True 3 True 4 True 5 True

The fuel cell is used to measure oxygen concentration. Piezo-electric crystals resonate at certain frequencies, which change when exposed to inhalational anaesthetics. Raman scattering is a change in the wavelength of light reflected from certain gas molecules, including volatile anaesthetics.

I.87 Regarding turbulent flow of gases in a breathing system:

1 False 2 False 3 False 4 False 5 True

When turbulent, flow is approximately proportional to the square root of the pressure. Decreasing the tubing diameter will decrease the flow, but there is not such a well-defined relationship as there is with laminar flow. In turbulent flow, density plays a greater role than viscosity. Turbulent flow is likely at Reynolds numbers of 2000 and above but is by no means certain. As gases heat up their density falls, decreasing the likelihood of turbulent flow.

I.88 100 mmHg pressure is approximately equal to:

1 True 2 False 3 False 4 False 5 True

100 kPa is atmospheric pressure, i.e. 1 bar or 14.5 psi or 133 cmH_2O. One torr is approximately equal to 1 mmHg.

I.89 Brainstem auditory evoked potentials (BAEPs):

1 True 2 False 3 True 4 True 5 True

I.90 Regarding the measurement of gastric intramucosal PCO_2:

1 True 2 False 3 False 4 True 5 True

II.1   In hyperparathyroidism, the following are typical:

1 Hypercalcaemia.
2 Low urinary calcium.
3 High serum phosphate.
4 No symptoms.
5 Osteitis fibrosis cystica.

II.2   Hypokalaemia is seen in:

1 Conn's syndrome.
2 Bartter's syndrome.
3 Cushing's syndrome.
4 Addison's disease.
5 Renal tubular acidosis.

II.3   Regarding oesophageal perforation:

1 Iatrogenic injury is the most common cause.
2 It should be considered in the presence of Meckler's triad.
3 It invariably produces symptoms within hours.
4 A normal initial chest X-ray reliably excludes the possibility of oesophageal perforation.
5 Timing of diagnosis is independent of subsequent morbidity and mortality.

II.4   Risk factors for adverse neurological outcome following cardiac surgery include:

1 Intraoperative hypertension (systolic arterial pressure > 180 mmHg for 10 minutes or more).
2 Intraoperative hypotension (systolic arterial pressure < 40 mmHg during cardiopulmonary bypass or < 80 mmHg for 10 minutes or more).
3 Congestive cardiac failure on the day of surgery.
4 Presence of peripheral vascular disease.
5 Age.

II.5   A patient with sickle cell disease:

1 Is susceptible to streptococcal infections.
2 Presenting for major elective surgery should be transfused to achieve an HbS level less than 30%.
3 Has a single point mutation resulting in abnormal α-globulin molecules.

4   With an alveolar–arterial oxygen gradient of more than 30 mmHg predicts the need for exchange transfusion in acute chest syndrome.

5   Should take folic acid supplements.

II.6   Regarding thyroid disease:

1   Hyperthyroidism is more prevalent in females than males.

2   Amiodarone can cause either hyper- or hypothyroidism.

3   The most common cause of goitre in developed countries is iodine deficiency.

4   Triiodothyronine (T_3) brings about its actions via cell surface receptor activation.

5   Hypercalcaemia is a recognized complication following thyroidectomy.

II.7   In variegate porphyria:

1   Aminolaevulinic acid is found in the urine.

2   Faecal porphyrins are only present during an acute attack.

3   Carbohydrate restriction is useful in the treatment of an acute attack.

4   Cutaneous bullae may occur on exposure to sunlight.

5   There is a deficiency of protoporphyrin oxidase.

II.8   Regarding atrial fibrillation and its treatment:

1   Thyrotoxicosis is the most common cause of atrial fibrillation.

2   The 'y' descent of the jugular venous pulse is obliterated.

3   According to the Vaughan Williams classification, propafenone is a class 1a drug.

4   The combination of digoxin and β-blockers should be avoided.

5   Direct current cardioversion is the best method of managing acute onset atrial fibrillation.

II.9   Presentation of a pituitary tumour may include:

1   Non-specific headache.

2   Infertility.

3   Acromegaly.

4   Epilepsy.

5   Third cranial nerve palsy.

II.10   Cushing's syndrome classically produces:

1   'Buffalo' obesity.

2   Hyponatraemia.

3   Hyperkalaemia.
4   Postural hypotension.
5   Buccal pigmentation.

II.11   The Wolff–Parkinson–White syndrome:

1   Has an incidence of 1.5% of the population.
2   Is characterized by a long P–R interval and a delta wave.
3   Is complicated by atrial fibrillation and atrioventricular tachycardia.
4   Can be treated with digoxin as a first-line therapeutic drug.
5   Needs catheter ablation in those at high risk for ventricular fibrillation.

II.12   Regarding thyroidectomy:

1   Complications occur more frequently during procedures for recurrent goitre.
2   Retrosternal enlargement of the thyroid can be asymptomatic.
3   Unintentional parathyroidectomy occurs in less than 1% of thyroidectomies.
4   The incidence of permanent unilateral vocal cord paralysis occurs in approximately 3%.
5   Repeat surgery for haemorrhage is required for 1–2% of cases.

II.13   Regarding phaeochromocytoma:

1   It is associated with von Recklinghausen's disease (neurofibromatosis).
2   It is diagnosed by measuring free catecholamines in a 24-hour urine collection.
3   Preoperative pharmacological control of arterial pressure is achieved primarily by β-adrenoceptor blockade.
4   Perioperative epidural blockade is absolutely contraindicated.
5   Persistent postoperative hypotension may occur.

II.14   The following may be typically found in tricyclic antidepressant poisoning:

1   Convulsions.
2   Coma.
3   Ataxia.
4   Dysrhythmia.
5   Jaundice.

II.15   Regarding pulmonary embolus:

1   Usually presents with severe retrosternal chest pain.
2   Dyspnoea, tachycardia and pleuritic pain are common on presentation.
3   ECG may show S1, qIII and T inversion in lead III.
4   Is frequently missed in the post-operative period.
5   Hypoxaemia is a consistent feature.

II.16   Regarding obesity:

1   It causes a fall in lung compliance.
2   The functional residual capacity (FRC) and residual volume (RV) fall significantly.
3   It is an independent risk factor for ischaemic heart disease.
4   It prolongs the elimination half-life of thiopentone.
5   Glomerular filtration rate and renal clearance increase.

II.17   Fasting for longer than 24 hours is associated with:

1   Hypoglycaemia.
2   Increased hepatic glycogenolysis.
3   Increased hepatic gluconeogenesis.
4   Increased protein catabolism.
5   Increased muscle gluconeogenesis.

II.18   The secretion of the following increases as part of the stress response to surgery:

1   Somatotrophin.
2   Prolactin.
3   Arginine vasopressin.
4   Triiodothyronine.
5   β-Endorphin.

II.19   Amiodarone:

1   Causes a widening of the QRS complex.
2   Can only be given parenterally.
3   Potentiates the effects of warfarin.
4   Produces pulmonary toxicity only after prolonged use.
5   Is indicated in the treatment of torsade de pointes.

II.20 In the treatment of tuberculosis (TB):

1 Respiratory TB requires treatment for a total period of 6 months.
2 Treatment of respiratory infection can commence without a positive sputum culture.
3 A different treatment regime is given to pregnant patients.
4 Side effects include peripheral neuropathy.
5 Rifampicin can be given intravenously.

II.21 The sciatic nerve:

1 Is formed by the anterior rami of S1–S4.
2 Lies over the quadratus femoris as it leaves the pelvis.
3 Provides sensation to the medial side of the ankle.
4 Can be blocked at the knee.
5 Terminates as the saphenous nerve.

II.22 Regarding the diaphragm:

1 It receives sensory supply from the last six intercostal nerves.
2 It is traversed by the oesophagus at the level of the eighth thoracic vertebral body.
3 It does not move during quiet respiration.
4 Congenital diaphragmatic herniae through the foramen of Morgagni are more common than those through the foramen of Bochdalek.
5 Congenital diaphragmatic herniae are more common on the left side.

II.23 Reflex sympathetic dystrophy (complex regional pain syndrome type 1):

1 Usually follows major trauma.
2 May occur in a patient with no history of trauma.
3 Is associated with pain in the distribution of one or more dermatomes.
4 Often results in a tender extremity.
5 Is common after cerebrovascular accidents.

II.24 The following may trigger malignant hyperthermia:

1 Pancuronium.
2 Ketamine.
3 Prilocaine.
4 Temazepam.
5 Atropine.

II.25 **Regarding the physiology of thermoregulation:**

1 Peripheral temperature receptors may also respond to non-thermal stimuli.
2 Peripheral receptors can respond to both cold and warm.
3 Peripheral cold sensation is transmitted by type A-delta nerve fibres.
4 Central cold receptors predominate over peripheral ones.
5 Central control of thermoregulation occurs primarily in the anterior thalamus.

II.26 **Suxamethonium can be used safely in:**

1 Patients with preoperative hyperkalaemia.
2 Patients exhibiting renal failure with normal preoperative serum potassium in the absence of associated neuropathy.
3 Repeated doses to patients with renal failure and a normal preoperative serum potassium.
4 Patients with uraemic polyneuropathy.
5 Repeated doses to patients with uraemic polyneuropathy.

II.27 **Ondansetron:**

1 Is a selective serotonin type 2 receptor.
2 Exerts no dopaminergic effects.
3 Effectively treats spinal/epidural morphine-induced pruritus.
4 Is recommended for use in breast-feeding mothers.
5 Causes flushing in some patients.

II.28 **Regarding desflurane:**

1 It has a blood:gas partition coefficient of 0.86.
2 Irritation of the airway during induction of anaesthesia can be reduced by increasing humidification of inspired gases.
3 It has better recovery characteristics than propofol.
4 Smoking increases the incidence of adverse airway events during desflurane anaesthesia.
5 Abstaining from smoking for 10 days prior to anaesthesia reduces adverse airway events during desflurane anaesthesia.

II.29 **Causes of loss of consciousness following spinal anaesthesia for Caesarean section include:**

1 Aortocaval compression.
2 Epileptic seizure.
3 Hypoxaemia.

4 Hypoglycaemia.

5 Hypotension.

II.30   Regarding heparin:

1 Low molecular weight heparin inhibits platelet function.

2 Unfractionated heparin inhibits platelet function.

3 Osteoporosis may occur with long-term low molecular weight heparin use.

4 Heparin-induced thrombocytopenia may occur with low molecular weight heparin therapy.

5 Low molecular weight heparin contains fewer mean saccharide units per molecule.

II.31   With regard to intraocular pressure:

1 It is required to maintain the shape of the eye.

2 Its control depends on the rate of inflow and outflow of aqueous.

3 It does not depend on the episcleral venous pressure.

4 It may be under hereditary influence.

5 The use of ketamine is associated with a decrease in pressure.

II.32   The following are true of the venous drainage of the heart:

1 The majority of the venous drainage is through the coronary sinus.

2 The coronary sinus drains into the great cardiac vein.

3 The venae cordis minimi drain into the right atrium.

4 The right marginal vein drains the lower border of the heart.

5 Veins rarely accompany the coronary arteries.

II.33   Off-pump coronary bypass (OPCAB) surgery is contraindicated:

1 When there is cardiomegaly.

2 In the presence of poor left ventricular function.

3 In the presence of fast atrial fibrillation.

4 In patients with calcified coronary arteries.

5 In the elderly (over 70 years).

II.34   With regard to adult epiglottitis:

1 It is seldom as severe as in children.

2 A conservative approach is advocated.

3 It is usually caused by *Haemophilus* influenzae type B.

4   Stridor and dyspnoea are unhelpful in predicting loss of the airway.

5   Bag and mask ventilation may protect the airway until intubation is achieved.

II.35   Regarding rapacurium:

1   It is within 10% of the efficacy of succinylcholine for rapid-sequence induction techniques.

2   It leads to an increased heart rate after induction.

3   At a dose of 2.5 mg kg^{-1} it has respiratory complications in nearly 20% of patients.

4   Smoking does not affect the frequency of respiratory complications.

5   It can safely be recommended as an alternative to succinylcholine.

II.36   Intracranial aneurysms:

1   Usually occur on the circle of Willis.

2   Are usually congenital.

3   10% occur in the vertebrobasilar system.

4   Rarely rupture if less than 5 mm in diameter.

5   Most commonly present before the age of 35 years.

II.37   From the pharmacokinetic point of view, Clevidipine:

1   Is an ultra-short-acting calcium channel antagonist.

2   Is metabolized largely by esterases within blood.

3   Has significant pulmonary extraction.

4   Probably has a temperature-dependent metabolism.

5   By infusion, reaches steady state within 2 minutes.

II.38   In aortic stenosis:

1   Anatomical restriction of the outflow tract limits cardiac output.

2   Valvular aortic stenosis often has a long asymptomatic phase.

3   Angina is the commonest presenting symptom.

4   Syncope is unusual.

5   If asymptomatic it does not cause problems with anaesthesia.

II.39   The haemolysis – elevated liver enzymes – low platelets (HELLP) syndrome:

1   Excludes hyperbilirubinaemia as a diagnostic criterion.

2   May present with nausea and vomiting.

3   Is usually associated with hypertension.

4 May present post partum.

5 Rarely requires platelet transfusion when the count is below $100 \times 10^9 \, l^{-1}$.

II.40   Concerning haemoglobin:

1 1.39 ml of oxygen can combine with a gram of haemoglobin.

2 2,3-DPG increases the amount of oxygen that haemoglobin can carry.

3 2,3-DPG concentration is well maintained in stored blood.

4 Cyanosis is more readily seen in anaemic patients.

5 Oxygen has one-tenth the affinity for haemoglobin as carbon monoxide.

II.41   Cardiac output is increased by:

1 Increased venous tone.

2 Inspiration.

3 Positive end-expiratory pressure (PEEP).

4 Lignocaine.

5 Halothane.

II.42   Sympathetic stimulation causes:

1 Contraction of the gall-bladder.

2 Glucose release from the liver.

3 Reduced cardiac output.

4 Reduced sweating.

5 Increased peristalsis.

II.43   The following drugs are safe in porphyria:

1 Thiopentone.

2 Morphine.

3 Aspirin.

4 Vecuronium.

5 Methohexitone.

II.44   Concerning transurethral resection (TUR) syndrome:

1 It consists of haemolysis and hypernatraemia.

2 Glycine is used in irrigation fluid to allow diathermy.

3 Glycine is an excitatory neurotransmitter.

4 Low intravesicular pressures abolish absorption.

5 Ethanol excretion can be used as a measure of fluid absorption.

II.45 Acupuncture:

1 Stimulates A-delta nerve fibres.
2 Releases endogenous opioids.
3 Causes increases in serum serotonin.
4 Causes increased ACTH release.
5 Has been shown to reduce postoperative nausea and vomiting.

II.46 Regarding chronic back pain:

1 The nerve to the facet joint is a mixed (sensory and motor) peripheral nerve.
2 Epidural steroids have been proven to be of benefit in acute back pain.
3 Epidurals have been shown to be of benefit in chronic back pain.
4 Epidural steroids are thought to work at steroid receptors in the spinal cord.
5 It responds to surgery in approximately 30% of cases.

II.47 The functional residual capacity:

1 Is the volume remaining in the lungs after a maximal expiration.
2 Is increased in emphysema.
3 Is increased in pregnancy.
4 Can be measured by spirometry.
5 Is approximately 2 litres in the normal adult.

II.48 Postoperative hypertension:

1 May result in myocardial infarction.
2 Is best treated by the administration of a β-blocker.
3 Is prevented by continuing concurrent antihypertensive medication up to the time of surgery.
4 Is prevented by continuing concurrent antihypertensive medication during the perioperative period.
5 May be relieved by catheterization of the bladder.

II.49 During mechanical ventilation:

1 Functional residual capacity is decreased.
2 Ventilation is evenly distributed throughout the lung.
3 $V_D:V_T$ ratio falls.

4   The reading on the ventilator pressure gauge reflects alveolar pressure.

5   Cardiac output is always reduced.

II.50   **The rate of diffusion of a gas across the alveolar–capillary membrane is affected by:**

1   The difference in partial pressure between the gas in the alveoli and that dissolved in the blood.

2   The thickness of the membrane.

3   The partial pressure of nitrogen in the inspired gas mixture.

4   Hyperventilation.

5   The introduction of nitrous oxide into the inspired gas mixture.

II.51   **If a child who has had respiratory distress syndrome at birth presents some months later for an inguinal hernia repair:**

1   The end-tidal CO_2 can be used with confidence to estimate the arterial CO_2.

2   It is more likely to be a male child.

3   Prophylactic antibiotics will be appropriate.

4   It will usually accept a larger than anticipated endotracheal tube.

5   It should be given large doses of opiates to suppress the stress response.

II.52   **Myocardial infarction in the postoperative period:**

1   Is most likely in the first 24 hours postoperatively.

2   Can be predicted reliably from preoperative overnight pulse oximetry.

3   Is less likely if β-adrenergic blockade is continued perioperatively.

4   Is associated with first-degree heart block seen on ECG.

5   Is less likely if surgery is delayed for 3 months after a previous myocardial infarction.

II.53   **Physiological haemostasis is a particular problem in patients with impaired liver function so that:**

1   Conventional hypocoagulability testing is a useful measure of the quality of coagulation factors.

2   The thromboelastograph is especially helpful because it measures fibrinolysis as well as hypocoagulability.

3   Desmopressin is contraindicated during surgery because it promotes platelet adhesiveness.

4   Thrombotic dissolution occurs rapidly in the cirrhotic patient.

5   The platelet count should not fall below 70 000 during surgery.

II.54 **Sevoflurane:**

1   Is a halogenated diethyl ether.
2   Has a blood/gas solubility coefficient of 0.68.
3   Forms Compound A in the presence of moist soda lime.
4   Metabolism may be induced by barbiturates.
5   Metabolism may be induced by CYP2E1 inducers.

II.55 **Regarding the following antibiotics:**

1   Ciprofloxacin is a third-generation cephalosporin.
2   Amoxycillin contains clavulanic acid to improve bioavailability.
3   Gentamicin is active against anaerobic bacterial infections.
4   Cefuroxime is completely safe to use in a patient with a penicillin allergy.
5   Co-amoxiclav is active against β-lactamase-producing bacteria.

II.56 **Cardioplegia solutions:**

1   Contain local anaesthetic.
2   Stop the heart in systole.
3   Are administered at body temperature.
4   Contain physiological concentrations of potassium.
5   Have a pH of 9.

II.57 **With regard to the visual pathway:**

1   A lesion in the optic nerve will cause a unilateral blindness.
2   The nerve fibres from the optic chiasm synapse in the medial geniculate nuclei.
3   A lesion at the chiasm will cause a homonymous hemianopia.
4   Relays in the superior colliculi are involved in the control of eye movements.
5   A lesion in the optic radiation will lead to a bitemporal hemianopia.

II.58 **In the fetal circulation:**

1   The umbilical arteries arise from the external iliac arteries.
2   The umbilical arteries carry oxygenated blood.
3   The ductus venosus bypasses the liver and allows blood to enter the inferior vena cava.
4   10% of the fetal circulation traverses the pulmonary circulation.
5   The parallel nature of the fetal circulation is split equally between the placenta and the systemic vasculature.

II.59 Regarding bradycardia:

1 It is defined as a heart rate less than 60 bpm.

2 Sinus and junctional bradycardias are treated as one group.

3 It is rarely associated with an inferior myocardial infarction.

4 Haemodynamic compromise may occur at faster rates than 60 bpm if there is also left ventricular failure.

5 Pacing is likely to be required if the rate falls below 40 bpm.

II.60 Regarding the vagus (CrX) nerve:

1 Secretomotor supply rises from the floor of the fourth ventricle.

2 Taste sensation is modulated in the nucleus tractus solitarius.

3 The nucleus ambiguus is the motor nucleus of the vagus.

4 The rootlets of the nerve leave the medulla medial to the olive.

5 The vagus leaves the skull through the jugular foramen.

II.61 The following are potential adverse effects of cell-free haemoglobin solutions:

1 Hypotension secondary to vasodilatation.

2 Methaemoglobinaemia.

3 Platelet activation.

4 Increased susceptibility to infection.

5 Interference with pulse oximetry.

II.62 Spinal shock:

1 Is where there is no sensory or motor function below an identifiable level.

2 May last days or months.

3 Has unaltered spinal reflex activity.

4 Is followed by hyperactivity of the spinal reflexes, especially those with phasic responses.

5 Is complicated by exaggerated autonomic reflexes such as the stretch response to bladder distension.

II.63 Concerning disseminated intravascular coagulation (DIC):

1 Low levels of coagulation factors secure the diagnosis.

2 Treatment of the cause is less important than replacing clotting factors.

3 Product of fibrinolysis may cause myocardial depression.

4   It can be caused by leukaemia.

5   Abnormalities in the blood film may be seen.

II.64 Compared to low-frequency large-volume ventilation, high-frequency ventilation by any method:

1   Is more efficient because the V_D : V_T ratio increases with frequency.

2   Causes an increase in lung volume.

3   Consistently increases cardiac output.

4   Causes a reflex suppression of ventilatory drive.

5   The majority of CO_2 clearance occurs by direct alveolar ventilation.

II.65 In a patient with chest trauma the following are indications for ventilation:

1   Associated head injury.

2   Severe shock.

3   Greater than eight rib fractures in a patient over 65 years of age.

4   An a-ADO_2 of 10 kPa on room air.

5   An isolated flail segment.

II.66 The pulmonary artery occlusion pressure (PAOP) or 'wedge' pressure:

1   Is an estimate of the left ventricular end-diastolic pressure.

2   Is unreliable if it exceeds pulmonary artery diastolic pressure (PADP).

3   Waveform should be flat.

4   Resembles a venous waveform.

5   Is reliable if the tip of the pulmonary artery catheter is situated in West's Zone 1 conditions.

II.67 Typical features 8 hours after salicylate poisoning include:

1   Coma.

2   Tinnitus.

3   Sweating.

4   Respiratory alkalosis in adults.

5   Improved excretion of drug with forced acid diuresis.

II.68 The following are true of positive inotropes:

1   Dobutamine can be safely administered via a peripheral vein.

2   Enoximone acts at β_1-adrenoceptors.

3 Dopexamine inhibits neuronal reuptake of noradrenaline.
4 Dopamine has a greater effect on β_2 than β_1-adrenoceptors.
5 Isoprenaline has chronotropic but not inotropic actions.

II.69 **Regarding hospital-acquired infections:**

1 They occur in 10% of all ICU admissions.
2 They are directly related to the age of the patient.
3 They are related to poor hand-washing practice.
4 They are greatly exacerbated by endotracheal intubation.
5 Selective decontamination of the gut has proven benefits.

II.70 **Concerning the scoring systems used in ICU:**

1 Apache III is a simplified version of Apache II.
2 The greater the Apache score the better the prognosis.
3 Scoring systems are now capable of being used to direct individual patient management.
4 The Simplified Acute Physiology Score is derived from 17 variables.
5 A lung injury score of 3 is indicative of mild to moderate lung injury.

II.71 **Multiple organ failure:**

1 Is the most common cause of death in intensive care.
2 Septicaemia is the most common presentation.
3 Occurs when normal organ homeostasis cannot be maintained by the patient.
4 Is closely associated with cytokine release.
5 May only occur in one system.

II.72 **Regarding the use of antibiotics:**

1 Cost is an important factor in the choice of antibiotic.
2 Gram-negative bacteria are a major problem in ICU.
3 Resistant fungal sepsis in still uncommon.
4 Differentiation between infection and colonization is often very difficult.
5 Hospital antibiotic policies have little impact on the emergence of resistant organisms.

II.73 **Obstructive shock:**

1 Is common.
2 May be due to a pulmonary embolism.

3 Is seen in pericardial tamponade.
4 Occurs in a pneumothorax.
5 Only affects the right side of the heart.

II.74 **Type 2 respiratory failure:**

1 Leads to hypercapnia.
2 Is commonly caused by morbid obesity.
3 Is commonly caused by acute lung injury.
4 Rarely occurs as an acute progression from type 1 failure.
5 Occurs in patients with neuromuscular problems.

II.75 **The following 'initial' ventilator settings are appropriate:**

1 Respiratory rate of 15 breaths per minute.
2 An inspiratory flow rate of 60 l min^{-1}.
3 A positive end-expiratory pressure (PEEP) of 0.
4 Tidal volumes of 15 ml kg^{-1}.
5 An I:E ratio of 1:2.

II.76 **Regarding liver failure:**

1 It can be classified using the Child–Pugh system.
2 It is rarely caused by ischaemia.
3 Encephalopathy is associated with a normal intracranial pressure.
4 N-Acetylcysteine should be given prophylactically.
5 It may lead to an adult respiratory distress syndrome (ARDS)-like syndrome.

II.77 **Regarding sedation on ICU:**

1 Accumulation of active metabolites is a problem with the benzodiazepines.
2 The pethidine metabolite norpethidine is a CNS sedative.
3 Clearance of fentanyl after prolonged infusion is prolonged.
4 The Ramsay sedation scale has two levels of assessment.
5 Sedation usually provides adequate analgesia unless painful stimuli are imposed.

II.78 **Indications for neuromuscular blockade include:**

1 Patients with high oxygen requirements.
2 Acute intubation and stabilization.
3 Tetanus.

4   Inappropriately high respiratory drive.

5   Reduction of the rate of sedative agent administration.

II.79   **Abnormal grief reactions are more likely:**

1   In sudden medical deaths.

2   In paediatric cases.

3   In an unsupportive family.

4   In traumatic deaths.

5   If transplantation is requested.

II.80   **Regarding ethics:**

1   Autonomy is the right of self-determination.

2   Beneficence is the right to the best quality of care.

3   Justice is the balancing of resources between patients.

4   Non-maleficence limits the ability to withdraw care.

5   Withdrawal of treatment must be with the consent of a close relative.

II.81   **Entonox:**

1   Is the trade name for a 70:30 mixture of nitrous oxide and oxygen.

2   Cylinders are coloured blue with blue/white quartered shoulders.

3   Is supplied in cylinders at a pressure of 37 bar.

4   Cylinders must be kept above the pseudocritical temperature of −20°C.

5   If the cylinder temperature falls below the pseudocritical temperature, liquefaction of oxygen occurs.

II.82   **Regarding open and closed systems of gastric tonometry:**

1   Carbon dioxide accumulates within a closed system.

2   Cardiopulmonary bypass was used as a model of a closed system.

3   There is a greater increase in $PiCO_2$ under open system conditions.

4   Increased pHi associated with decreased arterial bicarbonate and steady $PiCO_2$ indicates reversible intestinal mucosal injury.

5   It is possible for open and closed system conditions to occur within a single patient.

II.83   **The following relate to the cerebral function monitor in an intensive care setting:**

1   It requires four recording electrodes.

2   The parietal area is used because of the underlying watershed blood supply.

3   A smoothly fluctuating pattern has a good prognosis.

4   An upward sawtooth pattern has a good prognosis.

5   Sedation should not be increased if it has reduced the baseline signal to below 5 V.

II.84   Diathermy:

1   Uses high frequencies to reduce the chance of electrocution.

2   Is less likely to interfere with pacemaker function if a unipolar system is used.

3   Can cause burns if the plate is improperly applied.

4   Uses a damped wave for coagulation.

5   Uses a pulsed wave for cutting.

II.85   Flow through tubes:

1   Are independent of viscosity if laminar.

2   Are independent of pressure if turbulent.

3   Are both laminar and turbulent in a rotameter.

4   Are inversely proportional to radius if laminar.

5   Are more likely to be laminar with rough-walled tubes.

II.86   Cylinders used to store anaesthetic gases:

1   Are filled to a greater extent in the tropics.

2   Are blue if used to store Entonox.

3   Are black with a black and white collar if used to store oxygen.

4   Are labelled with the weight of the full cylinder.

5   Are connected to the anaesthetic machine using a Bodok seal.

II.87   Regarding electric shock in the operating room:

1   To receive an electric shock, an individual must contact the electric circuit at two different points at different voltages.

2   The major risk is precipitation of ventricular fibrillation.

3   When electric current enters the body via the skin, it is termed microshock.

4   The severity of the shock received is inversely proportional to the individual's resistance.

5   Circuit breakers and fuses within electrical equipment are designed to protect individuals from significant shock.

II.88 Regarding the direct measurement of arterial pressure:

1 The catheter–transducer system should have a low natural resonant frequency.
2 The catheter–transducer system should be critically damped.
3 Overdamping produces overestimation of diastolic and mean arterial pressures.
4 The catheter in the system should be short, stiff and wide.
5 Air in the catheter produces an underdamped system.

II.89 With regard to jugular venous bulb saturation (SjvO$_2$) monitoring:

1 The normal range is greater than 80%.
2 Low values indicate cerebral hypoxia.
3 Rapid withdrawal of blood samples may result in inaccurate measurements.
4 Specificity of measurements is low.
5 Desaturation may follow cerebral vasospasm.

II.90 In blood gas analysis:

1 A voltage is applied between the anode and cathode of the Clark electrode.
2 Actual bicarbonate is a measured value.
3 Standard bicarbonate is a derived value.
4 pH is a derived value.
5 The Severinghaus electrode measures carbon dioxide tension by means of a change in pH.

II.1   In hyperparathyroidism, the following are typical:

1 True   2 False   3 False   4 True   5 True

Urinary calcium excretion increases as serum calcium rises. Serum phosphate levels are inversely proportional to serum calcium. The majority of patients are asymptomatic. Osteitis fibrosis cystica is a unique manifestation of hyperparathyroidism where the normal bone architecture is replaced with fibrous tissue.

(Potts JT. Diseases of the parathyroid gland and other hyper- and hypocalcaemic disorders. In: *Harrison's Principles of Internal Medicine*, 14th edition. McGraw-Hill, 1998: 2227–2247.)

II.2   Hypokalaemia is seen in:

1 True   2 True   3 True   4 False   5 True

Hyperkalaemia occurs in the later stages of Addision's disease. Bartter's syndrome is a combination resulting in hypokalaemia, metabolic alkalosis and hyperreninaemia, hyperaldosteronism secondary to extracellular volume concentration and juxtaglomerular hyperplasia.

(Braunwald E, Fauci AS, Kasper DL et al. *Harrison's Principles of Internal Medicine*, 14th edition. McGraw-Hill, 1998.)

II.3   Regarding esophageal perforation:

1 True   2 True   3 False   4 False   5 False

II.4   Risk factors for adverse neurological outcome following cardiac surgery include:

1 False   2 False   3 False   4 False   5 True

II.5   A patient with sickle cell disease:

1 True   2 False   3 False   4 True   5 True

II.6   Regarding thyroid disease:

1 True   2 True   3 False   4 False   5 False

The most common cause of goitre in developed countries is autoimmune thyroid disease. Triiodothyronine interacts with nuclear receptors. Hypocalcaemia may occur secondary to parathyroid gland disruption.

II.7 | In variegate porphyria:

1 False   2 False   3 False   4 True   5 True

Variegate porphyria is due to a deficiency of the enzyme protoporphyrin oxidase. It combines many of the features of acute intermittent porphyria and cutaneous porphyria. Faecal porphyrins are present during latent periods as well as during acute attacks. Urinary porphyrins are not present. Treatment of an acute attacks includes carbohydrate loading, fluids and β-blockers.

II.8 | Regarding atrial fibrillation and its treatment:

1 False   2 False   3 False   4 False   5 True

II.9 | Presentation of a pituitary tumour may include:

1 True   2 True   3 True   4 True   5 True

II.10 | Cushing's syndrome classically produces:

1 True   2 False   3 False   4 False   5 False

II.11 | The Wolff–Parkinson–White syndrome:

1 False. It is 0.015%.
2 False. It has a short P–R interval and a delta wave.
3 True
4 False. It can increase the risk of ventricular fibrillation.
5 True

II.12 | Regarding thyroidectomy:

1 True   2 True   3 False   4 False   5 False

II.13 Regarding phaeochromocytoma:

1 True   2 True   3 False   4 False   5 False

II.14 The following may be typically found in tricyclic antidepressant poisoning:

1 True   2 True   3 False   4 True   5 False

Tricyclic antidepressants block the uptake of monoamines in adrenergic and tryptaminergic nerve endings in the brain. Many also have significant anticholinergic properties. The direct effect of the drugs on cell membranes is obviously greater in overdose, and particularly affects the heart. Initial symptoms are usually anticholinergic.

II.15 Regarding pulmonary embolism:

1 False   2 True   3 True   4 True   5 False

Dyspnoea, tachycardia and pleuritic pain present most frequently. Hypoxia is frequently present. However, a normal arterial PO_2 is seen in a quarter of patients.

II.16 Regarding obesity:

1 True   2 False   3 True   4 True   5 True

II.17 Fasting for longer than 24 hours is associated with:

1 False   2 False   3 True   4 True   5 False

II.18 The secretion of the following increases as part of the stress response to surgery:

1 True   2 True   3 True   4 False   5 True

II.19 Amiodarone:

1 True   2 False   3 True   4 False   5 False

The electrophysiological effects of amiodarone are complex and incompletely understood. Its main effect seems to be prolongation of action potential and refractory period duration, i.e. Class 3 in the Vaughan Williams classification. However, depending on the route and duration of use it may also possess effects from Classes 1, 2 and 4. It also has non-competitive α- and β-blocking properties. The class effects result in a prolonged Q–T interval but a normal QRS complex. It can be given orally and intravenously, both routes requiring loading doses. Amiodarone potentiates the actions of digoxin, heparin and oral anticoagulants. It has many side effects, including pulmonary toxicity, which may take one of two forms. Either an acute process resembling adult respiratory distress syndrome or a chronic process resembling an infectious pneumonitis can occur. The overall incidence of pulmonary toxicity is 5–10%. Amiodarone is contraindicated in the treatment of torsade de pointes.

II.20	In the treatment of tuberculosis (TB):
1 True	2 True	3 False	4 True	5 True

II.21	The sciatic nerve:
1 False	2 True	3 False	4 True	5 False

The sciatic nerve is the largest branch of the sacral plexus, being formed by the anterior rami of L4–S3. It leaves the pelvis via the greater sciatic notch, crossing the posterior aspect of the ischium on quadratus femoris and adductor magnus. It can be blocked in the buttock, the upper thigh and the popliteal fossa. Sensation to the medial side of the ankle is provided by the saphenous nerve, the terminal branch of the femoral nerve.

II.22	Regarding the diaphragm:
1 True	2 False	3 False	4 False	5 True

The oesophagus passes through the diaphragm at the level of the tenth thoracic vertebral body. Eighty percent of congenital diaphragmatic herniae occur through the foramen of Bochdalek, most commonly on the left.

II.23	Reflex sympathetic dystrophy (complex regional pain syndrome type 1):
1 False	2 True	3 False	4 True	5 True

Reflex sympathetic dystrophy, renamed complex regional pain syndrome type 1 by the International Association for the Study of Pain (IASP) in 1995, usually follows minor injury or surgery. The injury may be so slight that it is not remembered by the patient. It occurs in 12–25% of patients after acute brain injury or stroke. A tender extremity with mild swelling usually occurs.

II.24	The following may trigger malignant hyperthermia:

1 False	2 False	3 False	4 False	5 False

II.25	Regarding the physiology of thermoregulation:

1 True	2 False	3 True	4 False	5 False

II.26	Suxamethonium can be used safely in:

1 False	2 True	3 False	4 False	5 False

II.27	Ondansetron:

1 False	2 True	3 True	4 False	5 True

II.28	Regarding desflurane:

1 False	2 True	3 True	4 True	5 True

II.29	Causes of loss of consciousness following spinal anaesthesia for Caesarean section include:

1 True	2 True	3 True	4 True	5 True

II.30	Regarding heparin:

1 True	2 False	3 True	4 True	5 True

II.31	With regard to intraocular pressure:

1 True	2 True	3 True	4 True	5 False

Intraocular pressure in the general population appears to be under hereditary influence and is required to maintain the shape of the eye. It is a function of the differential rate of inflow and outflow of aqueous from the eye. It does not depend on the episcleral venous pressure. Ketamine increases intraocular pressure, unlike many intravenous anaesthetic agents.

II.32	The following are true of the venous drainage of the heart:
1 False	2 False	3 True	4 True	5 False

The majority of the venous drainage of the heart is via accompanying veins to the coronary arteries. They drain into the right atrium, as does the rest of the drainage. The coronary sinus has as tributaries the great, middle and small cardiac veins as well as the oblique and left posterior ventricular veins. Other drainage is through the venae cordis minimi and the anterior cardiac vein.

II.33	Off-pump coronary bypass (OPCAB) surgery is contraindicated:
1 True	2 False	3 True	4 True	5 False

The data for OPCAB does not support the suggestion that poor ventricular function and a reduced ejection fraction is a contraindication although cardiomegaly causes access difficulties. It may be the technique of choice in the elderly, especially if they have other risk factors such as renal impairment or prior stroke.

II.34	With regard to adult epiglottitis:
1 False	2 True	3 False	4 False	5 False

Adult epiglottitis is just as severe as in children although the causative organism is rarely identified, suggesting a viral cause. Rapid onset of stridor is one of the prime indicators that the airway is severely compromised and may be lost. Rapid-sequence induction has been recommended, with cricothyroid puncture equipment at hand, to avoid the problems with adult gaseous inductions, or the risk of bag and mask ventilation, which makes the obstruction worse.

(Ames WA, Ward VMM, Tranter RMD, Street M. Adult epiglottitis: an under-recognized, life-threatening condition. *Br J Anaesth* 2000; 85: 795–797.)

II.35	Regarding rapacurium:
1 True	2 True	3 True	4 False	5 False

(Blobner M, Mirakhur RK, Wierda JMK et al. Rapacurium 2.0 or 2.5 mg/kg for rapid-sequence induction: comparison with succinylcholine 1.0 mg/kg. *Br J Anaesth* 2000; 85: 724–731.)

II.36	Intracranial aneurysms:
	1 True 2 False 3 False 4 True 5 False

II.37	From the pharmacokinetic point of view, Clevidipine:
	1 True 2 False 3 False 4 True 5 True

Clevidipine is a new ultra-short-acting vasodilating calcium channel antagonist with an ester side chain that has been developed for intravenous administration. It rapidly equilibrates and does reach steady-state kinetics within 2 minutes when given by infusion. It is largely metabolized by extravascular esterases and has almost no pulmonary extraction. It appears to have a slower elimination during hypothermic bypass that is not due to haemodilution.

(Vuylsteke A, Milner Q, Ericsson H et al. Pharmocokinetics and pulmonary extraction of Clevidipine: a new vasodilating ultrashort-acting dihydropyridine during cardiopulmonary bypass. *Br J Anaesth* 2000; 85: 683–689.)

II.38	In aortic stenosis:
	1 True 2 True 3 True 4 False 5 True

Anaesthesia is usually uncomplicated if the patient is asymptomatic and does not have cardiomegaly.

II.39	The haemolysis – elevated liver enzymes – low platelets (HELLP) syndrome:
	1 False 2 True 3 False 4 True 5 True

II.40	Concerning haemoglobin:
	1 True 2 False 3 False 4 False 5 False

II.41	Cardiac output is increased by:
	1 True 2 True 3 False 4 False 5 False

II.42 Sympathetic stimulation causes:

1 False   2 True   3 False   4 False   5 False

II.43 The following drugs are safe in porphyria:

1 False   2 True   3 True   4 True   5 False

II.44 Concerning transurethral resection (TUR) syndrome:

1 False   2 True   3 False   4 False   5 True

II.45 Acupuncture:

1 True   2 True   3 True   4 True   5 True

II.46 Regarding chronic back pain:

1 False   2 True   3 False   4 False   5 True

II.47 The functional residual capacity:

1 False   2 True   3 False   4 False   5 True

II.48 Postoperative hypertension:

1 True   2 False   3 False   4 False   5 True

The best treatment is that of the identified cause. Hypertension can occur with a normal or even low heart rate and a vasodilator would be more suitable. The incidence of postoperative hypertension is greatest in those already suffering from hypertension and the degree and incidence can be reduced by continuing medication, but this does not eliminate the problem. Oral medication is seldom possible after major surgery and although systemic administration reduces the risk of postoperative hypertension it does not abolish it. A full bladder should always be considered as a cause for postoperative hypertension (or hypotension).

II.49   During mechanical ventilation:

1 True   2 False   3 False   4 False   5 False

Functional residual capacity reduction is probably due to a reduction in the tone of the diaphragm and shifts in blood volume between the thorax and abdomen. Ventilation is more evenly distributed during spontaneous breathing, but is preferentially distributed to the upper regions of the lung. The V_D rises due to a mismatch of ventilation and perfusion, and possibly due to bronchiolectasis. There is a progressive fall in pressure due to the compliance of the ventilator tubing and airway resistance. Cardiac output is generally reduced but in some cases of severe left ventricular failure output is improved by the reduction in left ventricular preload.

II.50   The rate of diffusion of a gas across the alveolar–capillary membrane is affected by:

1 True   2 True   3 False   4 False   5 True

At equilibrium nitrogen has no effect, whereas nitrous oxide causes the second gas effect and increases the diffusion gradient.

II.51   If a child who has had respiratory distress syndrome at birth presents some months later for an inguinal hernia repair:

1 False   2 True   3 True   4 False   5 False

If the child has bronchopleural dysplasia there may be a clinically significant difference between the end-tidal and arterial CO_2. There is a greater frequency in male children. Antibiotics are appropriate because these children have a higher than normal incidence of patent ductus arteriosus, with its risk of bacterial endocarditis. Intubation may be more difficult than anticipated because of subglottic stenosis from prolonged intubation and ventilation. They remain very sensitive to respiratory depression.

II.52   Myocardial infarction in the postoperative period:

1 False   2 False   3 True   4 False   5 True

Myocardial infarction is most likely from the second postoperative day onwards, but may occur at any time. Effective pain control may mask the warning anginal symptoms. Episodic hypoxaemia is associated with myocardial ischaemia, but is poorly predictive of infarction. β-Adrenergic blockade is protective against ischaemic event throughout the perioperative period.

| **II.53** | Physiological haemostasis is a particular problem in patients with impaired liver function so that: |

| 1 False | 2 True | 3 False | 4 True | 5 True |

Conventional tests are only quantitative and do not take the physiological status of the patient into account. The thromboelastograph, however, does measure the quality of the coagulation factors in the presence of abnormal physiological conditions. Desmopressin is effective in cardiopulmonary bypass surgery because of its platelet adhesive-enhancing properties, and it has a role in the operative management of patients with liver disease. Cirrhotic patients do appear to dissolve thromboses more rapidly, possibly because of increased fibrinolytic activity. Rapid, large volume transfusion to compensate for major blood loss leads to a dilutional coagulopathy that should be prevented by administering fresh frozen plasma and platelets. A value of 70 000 for platelets is appropriate.

| **II.54** | Sevoflurane: |

| 1 False | 2 True | 3 True | 4 False | 5 True |

Sevoflurane is a fluorinated methyl-isopropyl ether. Compound A is produced in small amounts in the presence of moist soda lime. Barbiturates do not induce sevoflurane metabolism.

| **II.55** | Regarding the following antibiotics: |

| 1 False | 2 False | 3 False | 4 False | 5 True |

Ciprofloxacin is a quinolone. Amoxycillin does not contain clavulanic acid, and has a spectrum of activity similar to ampicillin, with improved bioavailability. Gentamicin is inactive against anaerobes and some *Streptococcus* species. There is an approximate 10% risk of precipitating an allergic reaction with cefuroxime in penicillin-sensitive patients.

| **II.56** | Cardioplegia solutions: |

| 1 True | 2 False | 3 False | 4 False | 5 False |

Procaine is added as a membrane-stabilizing agent. Solutions contain 10–20 mmol l^{-1} of potassium and have a pH between 5.5 and 7.8. It is given cold, traditionally at 5 °C. cardiac arrest occurs in diastole.

| **II.57** | With regard to the visual pathway: |

| 1 True | 2 False | 3 False | 4 True | 5 False |

The main relays are in the lateral geniculate nuclei and lesions beyond here will cause a homonymous hemianopia. Those before will cause a bitemporal visual loss.

II.58	In the fetal circulation:

1 False	2 False	3 True	4 True	5 False

The umbilical arteries arise from the internal iliac arteries and carry deoxygenated blood to the placenta. The umbilical veins carry the oxygenated blood back. The ductus venosus shunts 50% of the returning blood directly into the inferior vena cava. The placenta/systemic split is approximately 60%/40%.

II.59	Regarding bradycardia:

1 True	2 True	3 False	4 True	5 False

One of the more common causes of a marked bradycardia is an inferior infarction. Pacing is indicated in bradycardias due to Mobitz type 2 atrioventricular (AV) block and third-degree (complete) AV block. In these patients atropine 1 mg is only a holding strategy until pacing can be organized and instituted.

II.60	Regarding the vagus (CrX) nerve:

1 True	2 True	3 True	4 False	5 True

There are three nuclei for the vagus, and the dorsal nucleus in the floor of the fourth ventricle is a mixed motor and sensory centre. The rootlets leave lateral to the olive and then fuse to form the longest of the cranial nerves, which leaves as a single trunk from the jugular foramen.

II.61	The following are potential adverse effects of cell-free haemoglobin solutions:

1 True	2 False	3 False	4 True	5 True

II.62	Spinal shock:

1 True	2 True	3 False	4 True	5 False

II.63	Concerning disseminated intravascular coagulation (DIC):

1 False	2 False	3 True	4 True	5 True

II.64 Compared to low-frequency large-volume ventilation, high-frequency ventilation by any method:

1 False   2 True   3 False   4 True   5 True

As the V_D: V_T ratio increases, the proportion of each breath available for alveolar ventilation decreases. Consequently the minute ventilation requirement increases with the frequency for all modes of high-frequency ventilation. Equally, the lung volume increases with high-frequency ventilation because the time available for expiration is short and the expiratory resistance is much greater than the inspiratory resistance. The increase is least for high-frequency oscillation and greatest for high-frequency positive pressure ventilation in flow generator mode. Circulatory effects are inconsistent. Ventilatory drive is suppressed with all modes of high-frequency ventilation and is thought to be due to the increase in lung volume. Direct alveolar ventilation accounts for most of the CO_2 elimination.

II.65 In a patient with chest trauma the following are indications for ventilation:

1 True   2 True   3 True   4 False   5 False

The presence of other injuries is often an indication to institute artificial ventilation and a head injury in particular is associated with a poor prognosis. The presence of a flail segment by itself is not an indication to institute ventilation but may be if associated with an underlying lung contusion. Flail segments are more common in the elderly because of their more brittle bones.

II.66 The pulmonary artery occlusion pressure (PAOP) or 'wedge' pressure:

1 True   2 True   3 False   4 True   5 False

The waveform resembles the left atrial pressure waveform. There should be a continuous column of blood between the catheter tip and left ventricle, i.e. West's Zone 3 conditions.

II.67 Typical features 8 hours after salicylate poisoning include:

1 False   2 True   3 True   4 True   5 False

Some patients are restless and confused but coma is rare. An initial respiratory acidosis may be superseded by a respiratory acidosis as a terminal effect. Metabolic acidosis usually predominates in children. Urinary excretion may be increased with *alkaline* diuresis.

II.68 The following are true of positive inotropes:

1 True   2 False   3 True   4 False   5 False

Enoximone is a phosphodiesterase inhibitor, acting at the cellular level, not via adrenoceptors. Dopamine has proportionately more activity at β_1 receptors. Isoprenaline increases both force and rate of myocardial contraction.

II.69 Regarding hospital-acquired infections:

1 False   2 True   3 True   4 True   5 False

The incidence is up to 20%, and a large variety of factors are involved, one of which is advancing age. The poor hand-washing practice by many medical and nursing staff is responsible for many of the infections. Artificial airways are very likely to lead to nosocomial infections, and selective decontamination has remained controversial, with minimal conclusive data on its effectiveness.

II.70 Concerning the scoring systems used in ICU:

1 False   2 False   3 False   4 True   5 False

Apache III is both complex and expensive, hence its limited use in the UK. The higher the score the greater the dysfunction and therefore the poorer the predicted outcome. There is no safe scoring system that can be used to direct patient care. A lung injury score of greater than 2.5 indicates severe lung injury or ARDS.

II.71 Multiple organ failure:

1 True   2 False   3 False   4 True   5 True

Septicaemia is no longer accepted as a diagnostic term, while others have been precisely defined (i.e. sepsis, septic shock or infection). The loss of organ homeostasis leading to organ failure occurs despite intervention. This intervention may be limited to fluid resuscitation or may involve advanced inotrope therapy. The definition of multiple organ dysfunction syndrome allows for one or more systems to be dysfunctional; respiratory failure is an example.

II.72 Regarding the use of antibiotics:

1 True   2 True   3 False   4 True   5 True

Gram-positive bacteria remain a major problem, with methicillin-resistant *Staphylococcus aureus* being almost endemic in UK intensive care units. Fungal infections are becoming more prevalent, and resistance is developing. The increase in resistant organisms is slowed by hospital antibiotic policies – where they are known and adhered to. There are increasing problems with resistance in gram negative organisms as well.

II.73	Obstructive shock:
	1 False 2 True 3 True 4 False 5 False

Obstructive shock is uncommon, and is due to either obstructed venous return or arterial outflow. The causes may be due to external pressure or directly from masses within the vessels. Rapid diagnosis is essential and life saving. *Tension* pneumothorax is probably one of the commonest causes and may be difficult to diagnose unless suspected and the clinical signs of hyper-resonance and reduced air entry sought.

II.74	Type 2 respiratory failure:
	1 True 2 True 3 False 4 False 5 True

Acute lung injury is more usually associated with type 1 failure. Type 1 can move rapidly to type 2 failure in intensive care, if there is evolution of the underlying cause – severe asthma for example.

II.75	The following 'initial' ventilator settings are appropriate:
	1 False 2 True 3 False 4 False 5 True

The most usual initial settings, which are then altered to individualize later ventilation, include: a frequency of 10 breaths per minute, a tidal volume of 10 ml kg^{-1}, a PEEP of 5 cmH$_2$O and an inspired oxygen concentration of 100%.

II.76	Regarding liver failure
	1 True 2 False 3 False 4 True 5 True

Ischaemia is believed to underlie many of the other causes of liver failure, and leads to global liver dysfunction. Encephalopathy is commonly associated with a raised intracranial pressure, and direct monitoring should be considered early. The hepatopulmonary syndrome resembles ARDS and, while the cause is not known, it may be a result of oedema or infection.

II.77 Regarding sedation on ICU:

1 True   2 False   3 True   4 True   5 False

Norpethidine is a proconvulsant drug and leads to CNS hyperexcitability. Sedation very rarely provides adequate analgesia and most scoring systems avoid the testing of the adequacy of analgesia.

II.78 Indications for neuromuscular blockade include:

1 True   2 True   3 True   4 True   5 False

Paralysis is usually used for short periods and for specific indications since effective sedation and analgesic methods have been developed. If it is needed, for instance to reduce respiratory drive or reduce oxygen consumption, it should be titrated to a monitored single visible twitch on a train-of-four stimulation. Caution is necessary because of drug accumulation.

II.79 Abnormal grief reactions are more likely:

1 False   2 False   3 True   4 True   5 False

Complicated family situations, with histories of estrangement or conflict, are likely to lead to abnormal reactions. Expected or medical deaths are less likely to lead to abnormal reactions, partly because the process of grieving has already started prior to death.

II.80 Regarding ethics:

1 True   2 False   3 True   4 False   5 False

Beneficence is related to our duty of care and to achieve the best we can. Justice may be seen to equate to the balancing of meagre resources to achieve the best for all patients. Non-maleficence, or avoiding harm, has to be balanced with beneficence as a risk/benefit analysis and may lead (as in futility) to alterations in the planned care. Consent is a matter for the doctor and the patient alone, unless an advanced directive nominates an advocate prior to the event.

II.81 Entonox:

1 False   2 True   3 False   4 False   5 True

Entonox is a 50:50 mixture of oxygen and nitrous oxide. Cylinder pressure is 137 bar. The pseudocritical temperature is −7°C. Below this temperature liquefaction of nitrous oxide occurs.

II.82	Regarding open and closed systems of gastric tonometry:

1 True   2 False   3 False   4 True   5 True

II.83	The following relate to the cerebral function monitor in an intensive care setting:

1 False   2 True   3 True   4 False   5 True

II.84	Diathermy:

1 True   2 True   3 True   4 True   5 False

II.85	Flow through tubes:

1 True   2 False   3 True   4 False   5 False

II.86	Cylinders used to store anaesthetic gases:

1 False   2 False   3 False   4 False   5 True

II.87	Regarding electric shock in the operating room:

1 True   2 True   3 False   4 True   5 False

Electric current entering through the skin is termed macroshock. Ohm's law dictates that current equals voltage divided by resistance. Increasing resistance (e.g. by wearing rubber shoes) lowers current flow. Circuit breakers and fuses are designed to prevent electrical fires. They typically interrupt power when the current exceeds 10 amperes; this is 100 times greater than that needed to produce ventricular fibrillation.

II.88	Regarding the direct measurement of arterial pressure:

1 False   2 False   3 False   4 True   5 False

The arterial waveform is a complex waveform. Fourier analysis reveals a fundamental wave (the pulse rate) and a series of harmonics of increasing frequency. The natural frequency of the system needs to be high to obtain accurate reproduction of these harmonics. Classically, systems are damped to 0.64 of critical (critical damping = no overshoot with stepwise change in pressure). Air in the catheter produces an overdamped system, resulting in underestimation of systolic pressure, overestimation of diastolic pressure and no change in mean arterial pressure.

II.89	With regard to jugular venous bulb saturation (SjvO$_2$) monitoring:

1 False	2 False	3 True	4 True	5 True

SjvO$_2$ is a measure of global hemispheric venous oxygen saturation. The normal value lies between 54% and 75%. A low value does not indicate hypoxia, but only an increase in oxygen extraction that may result in ischaemia if uncorrected. Up to 50% of desaturations may be false positives (i.e. specificity is low). Rapid withdrawal of blood samples may result in contamination of the sample with extracranial blood.

II.90	In blood gas analysis:

1 True	2 False	3 True	4 False	5 True

Blood gas analysers measure PCO$_2$, PO$_2$ and pH. All other values are derived. In the Severinghaus electrode diffusion of carbon dioxide into a bicarbonate solution causes a change in pH. As pH changes linearly with the logarithm of the carbon dioxide tension, the machine is calibrated in terms of PCO$_2$.

III.1   Causes of secondary hyperparathyroidism include:

1   Chronic renal failure.
2   Rickets.
3   Vitamin D deficiency.
4   Sarcoidosis.
5   Multiple myeloma.

III.2   Regarding multiple endocrine neoplasia type 1 (MEN 1):

1   It is an autosomal recessive familial cancer syndrome.
2   By the age of 40 years, greater than 95% of patients have hypercalcaemia.
3   Pituitary adenomas are the most common lesion in MEN 1.
4   It is associated with phaeochromocytoma.
5   It is associated with anterior pituitary tumours.

III.3   The following cause a raised serum creatine kinase concentration:

1   Hypothyroidism.
2   Myocardial infarction.
3   Hypertrophic obstructive cardiomyopathy.
4   Neuroleptic malignant syndrome.
5   Myasthenia gravis.

III.4   Phenoxybenzamine:

1   Is a competitive adrenoceptor antagonist.
2   Selectively blocks α_1-adrenoceptors.
3   Often causes tachycardia.
4   May decrease consciousness level.
5   Should not be given to patients receiving β-blockers.

III.5   The following may result in massive haemoptysis:

1   Goodpasture's syndrome.
2   Behçet's disease.
3   Wegener's granulomatosis.
4   Mitral stenosis.
5   Bronchiectasis.

III.6 Wegener's granulomatosis:

1 Usually presents between 25 and 50 years of age.
2 Never presents in childhood.
3 Pulmonary lesions are present in 95% of cases.
4 May induce spontaneous pneumothorax.
5 Is treated with third-generation cephalosporins.

III.7 Regarding inherited disorders of haemostasis:

1 Haemophilia A is an autosomal recessive condition.
2 Haemophilia B is observed in 5% of Ashkenazi Jews.
3 Von Willebrand's disease is an X-linked recessive condition.
4 Afibrinogenaemia is otherwise known as factor I deficiency.
5 Christmas disease (Haemophilia B) is caused by factor X deficiency.

III.8 Regarding familial periodic paralysis:

1 The inheritance pattern is that of an autosomal recessive.
2 The hypokalaemic form rarely affects breathing and swallowing.
3 The hypokalaemic form is severely affected if the serum potassium falls below 3.0 mmol l^{-1}.
4 The hyperkalaemic form often occurs while resting after exercise.
5 Arrhythmias are common in the normokalaemic paralysis patients.

III.9 Concerning renal function:

1 *para*-Aminohippuric acid (PAH) clearance measures glomerular filtration rate.
2 Inulin is filtered but not absorbed or excreted by the tubules.
3 20% of glomerular filtrate is absorbed in the proximal tubule.
4 The thin section of the loop of Henle is very metabolically active.
5 ADH controls water balance by its effect on the collecting duct.

III.10 Subarachnoid haemorrhage:

1 Is caused by atrioventricular malformations in 30% of cases.
2 Is caused by trauma in 20% of cases.
3 Is caused by aneurysm on the posterior part of the circle of Willis in 40% of cases.
4 Causes vasospasm, seen most commonly at 1 day post haemorrhage.
5 Rarely causes hyponatraemia.

III.11   Regarding atrial fibrillation and its treatment:

1 The optimum ventricular rate in chronic atrial fibrillation is 90 bpm.
2 Direct current cardioversion should not be used in atrial fibrillation of more than 48 hours duration without at least 8 weeks of anticoagulation.
3 The risk of systemic embolization after cardioversion in non-anticoagulated patients is around 1%.
4 Verapamil produces more hypotension than esmolol.
5 Transoesophageal echocardiography is useful in identifying patients, who may be safely cardioverted without anticoagulation.

III.12   The following clinical conditions produce a right-to-left shunt:

1 Lobar pneumonia.
2 Pulmonary embolism.
3 Fallot's tetralogy.
4 Post-ductal coarctation of the aorta.
5 Patent ductus arteriosus.

III.13   Haemoglobin A:

1 Is formed within erythrocytes.
2 Is the predominant form of haemoglobin in the adult.
3 Contains two α and two β polypeptide globin chains.
4 Binds 2,3-DPG more avidly than fetal haemoglobin.
5 Contains iron, which reversibly enters the ferric state when converting from deoxyhaemoglobin to oxyhaemoglobin.

III.14   The administration of magnesium may result in:

1 Shortening of the Q–T interval.
2 Potentiation of non-depolarizing neuromuscular block.
3 Tocolysis.
4 Bronchoconstriction.
5 Decreased forced vital capacity (FVC).

III.15   A long Q–T interval may occur with:

1 Hypothermia.
2 Hypercalcaemia.
3 Tricyclic antidepressant therapy.

4   Cerebral injury.

5   Digoxin.

III.16   **von Willebrand's disease:**

1   Is inherited as autosomal dominant.

2   Causes a prolonged prothrombin time.

3   Affected patients have a prolonged bleeding time.

4   Commonly results in haemarthrosis.

5   Treatment with desmopressin increases the platelet count.

III.17   **Features of hypothyroidism include:**

1   Menorrhagia.

2   Malar flush.

3   Absent ankle tendon reflexes.

4   Carpal tunnel syndrome.

5   Deafness.

III.18   **Regarding epiglottitis:**

1   It has a peak incidence between 6 and 18 months of age.

2   It usually causes a systemic upset in the child.

3   Intravenous access should be achieved prior to induction.

4   Intubation is seldom necessary beyond 12 hours.

5   It can occur in middle-aged adults.

III.19   **The following changes may be seen in animals after hepatectomy:**

1   Increased plasma glucose.

2   An increased plasma albumin:globulin ratio.

3   Increased plasma free fatty acids.

4   Decreased conversion of angiotensin 1 to angiotensin 2.

5   A fall in blood urea and an increase in plasma ammonia.

III.20   **Parathyroid hormone secretion increases in response to:**

1   A decrease in extracellular calcium concentration.

2   An increase in extracellular magnesium concentration.

3   An increase in vitamin D.

4   Propranolol.

5   Prednisolone.

III.21 The following are consistent with a diagnosis of neuroleptic malignant syndrome:

1 Pancuronium.
2 Ketamine.
3 Prilocaine.
4 Temazepam.
5 Atropine.

III.22 Dexmedetomidine:

1 Acts at α_1 receptors.
2 Increases anaesthetic requirements.
3 Acts principally through peripheral receptors.
4 Increases airway secretions.
5 Predisposes the patient to perioperative hypertension.

III.23 The following are associated with an increased risk of perioperative peripheral neuropathy of the corresponding nerves:

1 Supination of the forearm and ulnar nerve.
2 120° of elbow flexion and ulnar nerve.
3 120° of hip flexion and sciatic nerve.
4 120° of hip flexion and femoral nerve.
5 Padding over the lateral tibia and common peroneal nerve.

III.24 With regard to the oculocardiac reflex (OCR):

1 It leads to tachycardia.
2 It commonly occurs due to stretching of the extraocular muscles.
3 Retrobulbar anaesthesia blocks the efferent limb of this reflex.
4 Premedication with atropine does not have an effect on its incidence.
5 There is an association between the OCR and postoperative vomiting.

III.25 The following are true of the hypoglossal nerve (CrXII):

1 It is the motor supply to all of the intrinsic muscles of the tongue.
2 It is the motor supply to all the extrinsic muscles of the tongue.
3 It leaves the medulla as a series of rootlets before becoming a single trunk.
4 It leaves the skull through the jugular foramen.
5 It loops over the lingual artery at the angle of the jaw.

III.26 Ropivacaine:

1 Is an ester local anaesthetic.
2 Is of similar potency to bupivacaine.
3 Is a racemic mixture of isomers.
4 Has greater sensory compared to motor blockade than bupivacaine.
5 Has similar cardiotoxicity to bupivacaine.

III.27 Regarding postherpetic neuralgia:

1 It occurs in greater than 20% of cases.
2 It is defined as pain occurring after the disappearance of the vesicles.
3 It is common in those aged below 40 years.
4 Pain is felt bilaterally in the majority of patients.
5 Topical application of 'Clingfilm' is of use.

III.28 Physiological dead space:

1 Is greater than the anatomical dead space.
2 Remains constant with changes in tidal volume.
3 Increases following the induction of general anaesthesia.
4 Can be determined using a nitrogen washout technique.
5 Can be calculated from knowledge of the tidal volume, arterial pCO_2 and the mixed expired CO_2 concentration.

III.29 A 3.1 kg baby delivered at 39 weeks' gestation presents with respiratory distress due to a congenital diaphragmatic hernia 6 hours after birth:

1 The baby needs an emergency operation to repair the hernia.
2 Awake intubation prior to anaesthesia should be performed.
3 The theatre temperature should be maintained at 30°C.
4 A preoperative haematocrit of 55% implies that the baby is dehydrated.
5 Ideally arterial oxygen saturation should be maintained in the range 94–98%.

III.30 The following drugs are reduced by plasma cholinesterase (pseudocholinestrase):

1 *cis*-Atracurium.
2 Mivacurium.
3 Remifentanil.
4 Suxamethonium.
5 Amethocaine.

III.31 Functional residual capacity is increased by:

1 Tidal ventilation pre-oxygenation.
2 Placing an awake patient in an upright position from supine.
3 Positive end-expiratory pressure (PEEP).
4 Continuous positive-airways pressure (CPAP).
5 Asthma.

III.32 The IUPAC nomenclature of hydrocarbons:

1 Names the longest unbranched chain first.
2 Places the substituent groups in the middle of the name.
3 Then identifies the position of the groups.
4 This counting of position is such as to give the lowest number for these groups.
5 Is also applicable to fatty acids.

III.33 The cell cycle of a eukaryotic cell includes the following phases:

1 G_0 – a period of routine metabolic activity.
2 G_1 – cell growth.
3 G_2 – DNA replication.
4 M – mitosis or meiosis.
5 S – cell death.

III.34 The following are true in patients with untreated hypertension:

1 15% of cases have a specific aetiological factor.
2 A systolic pressure greater than 200 mmHg on three separate occasions should be treated.
3 A diastolic pressure greater than 90–109 mmHg on three separate occasions should be treated.
4 A systolic pressure of 160–190 mmHg should be checked monthly if there is no other medical indication.
5 Malignant hypertension is defined as a diastolic pressure greater than 140 mmHg.

III.35 The following changes occur in the nervous system with ageing alone:

1 Increased myelination of nerves.
2 Decrease in neurotransmitter synthesis.
3 Reduction in the number of synapses.

4   Maintained autonomic function.

5   Presbycusis.

III.36   In Hirschsprung's disease:

1   The prime defect is in the small gut.

2   The cause is a failure of migration of neuroblasts *in utero*.

3   Central hypoventilation commonly occurs in these patients.

4   Vomiting is a particular risk on induction of anaesthesia.

5   There is a female preponderance.

III.37   Halothane hepatitis:

1   Type 1 liver dysfunction occurs in 20% of patients.

2   Type 2 liver dysfunction occurs in 1 in 37 000 exposures.

3   Type 1 is due to localized hepatic hypoxia.

4   Type 2 is due to reductive metabolites.

5   Type 2 follows previous exposure in 50% of cases.

III.38   Etomidate:

1   Is an imidazole.

2   Is prepared in 20% propylene glycol.

3   Has a pH of 7.6.

4   Has an incidence of hypersensitivity of 1:30 000.

5   Has a therapeutic ratio ($LD_{50}:ED_{50}$) of 30.

III.39   Active transport across a cell membrane:

1   Occurs against a concentration gradient up to 10:1.

2   Is specific for molecular types.

3   Is responsible for the uptake of iodine into the thyroid.

4   Is the major system for the transport of sugars in the body.

5   May allow competitive transport of drugs such as adrenergic blockers.

III.40   Regarding sterilization:

1   It is the killing of all infected matter, including the most resistant organisms and spores.

2   For autoclaving it is dependent on temperature alone.

3   Dry heat is unsuitable for glass equipment.

4 Gamma radiation is the usual method of sterization for hospital reusable items.

5 Face masks are a semi-critical item and only require disinfection.

III.41   **The clotting factors' common names are as follows:**

1 Factor II is thrombin.

2 Factor VI is proaccelerin.

3 Factor IX is Christmas factor.

4 Factor X is glass factor.

5 Factor XIII is fibrin.

III.42   **Concerning suxamethonium apnoea:**

1 Plasma cholinesterase is also involved in the metabolism of morphine.

2 DNA analysis techniques have replaced dibucaine testing.

3 Onset of relaxation is normal.

4 It may be effectively treated by administering fresh frozen plasma.

5 The breakdown product succinyl monocholine is inactive.

III.43   **Concerning gross obesity:**

1 The standard operating table in the UK will safely support up to 35 stone (approximately 220 kg).

2 Arterial blood gas estimation is normal when corrected for age.

3 Polycythaemia is a normal finding in the very obese.

4 Invasive monitoring is advisable for most procedures.

5 An awake intubation should always be considered.

III.44   **Considering regional anaesthesia in the near-term obstetric patient:**

1 Hypotension should be treated by ephedrine because it has the least effect on the fetus.

2 Aortocaval compression is less problematical than if a general anaesthetic is used.

3 The volume of local anaesthetic needed to achieve blockade is reduced because of epidural venous congestion.

4 A block from T10 to S5 is adequate for a forceps delivery.

5 Signs of blood loss during Caesarean section will be masked under regional anaesthesia.

III.45 **With regard to opioid receptors:**

1 There are four opioid receptors.
2 There are subtypes for mu receptors.
3 They promote potassium inflow.
4 They inhibit voltage-gated calcium channels.
5 Analgesia is produced by activation of any of the opioid receptors.

III.46 **Considering a patient with jaundice:**

1 Clinical assessment will lead to a diagnosis in over 80% of patients.
2 Liver function tests indicate abnormal synthetic function of the liver.
3 Unconjugated bilirubin leading to jaundice occurs in up to 5% of the population.
4 A bilirubin over 20 μmol l^{-1} is capable of producing clinically recognizable jaundice.
5 γ-Glutamyl transpeptidase is a sensitive marker of enzyme induction.

III.47 **Concerning adhesion molecules:**

1 Cadherins are cell surface adhesion molecules.
2 Cadherins mediate cell growth and differentiation.
3 Integrins are glycoproteins that mediate intracellular interactions.
4 Selectins slow leukocytes and promote their adhesion to endothelium.
5 Anaesthetic agents have little effect on adhesion.

III.48 **Regarding arterial tourniquets:**

1 They are safe in sickle trait.
2 They should be placed where there is enough muscle bulk to protect underlying nerves.
3 Inflation times above 1 hour should be avoided.
4 Metabolic breakdown products accumulate and lead to acidosis.
5 The cuff pressure should be 250 mmHg in the lower limb.

III.49 **Regarding Apert's syndrome:**

1 It is an autosomal dominant disorder.
2 It is associated with a midfacial hypoplasia.
3 There is a 20% incidence of congenital cardiac defects.
4 Major cervical anomalies are common.
5 Raised intracranial pressure is rarely a problem.

III.50 With regard to intracranial aneurysms:

1 Basilar territory aneurysms occur in less than 5% of patients.
2 The commonest site is the anterior cerebral artery.
3 Aneurysms rarely rupture until they are over 5 mm in diameter.
4 A Hunt and Hess grade of 1 has a 95% chance of survival after 21 days.
5 Cerebral vasospasm occurs in up to 50% of patients with a subarachnoid haemorrhage.

III.51 Regarding dexamethasone and postoperative nausea and vomiting:

1 Dexamethasone is a rapidly acting anti-emetic.
2 It is effective at a dose of 2 mg.
3 Prolonged efficacy (up to 24 hours) occurs.
4 Dexamethasone 8 mg intravenously can cause genital discomfort and hyperaemia.
5 It reduces PCA–morphine-induced nausea and vomiting from 50–60% to 20%.

III.52 Concerning the basic mechanisms of anaesthesia:

1 Subanaesthetic concentrations of volatile anaesthetics suppress learning.
2 Volatile anaesthetics are usually in the range of solubility parameter of 10–11.
3 General anaesthetics all work at the $GABA_a$ receptor site.
4 Anaesthetic-sensitive ligand-gated ion channels have been described using X-ray crystallography.
5 Protein binding sites for general anaesthetics are mainly membrane based.

III.53 Concerning Parkinson's disease and anaesthesia:

1 Parkinson's disease affects 1% of the elderly population.
2 Symptoms become apparent after 50% of dopaminergic neurones are lost.
3 It is primarily a disorder of voluntary motor control.
4 Treatment regimens may be safely withheld during the perioperative period.
5 Apomorphine may be used parenterally for treatment if oral medication is withheld.

III.54 Concerning neuropathic pain:

1 All neuropathic pain syndromes have a defined lesion in the nervous system.
2 It is estimated to account for 25% of all referrals to pain clinics.
3 Allodynia is pathognomonic of neuropathic pain.

4   Neuropathic pain may be evoked or spontaneous.

5   Nerve growth factors have a major role in the prevention of diabetic neuropathy.

III.55   Concerning myasthenia gravis:

1   Thymic disease occurs in most people with myasthenia gravis.

2   Edrophonium 10 mg i.v. remains the standard diagnostic test.

3   It affects 1:1000 of the population.

4   A forced vital capacity of below 3 litres is a poor sign of respiratory function.

5   Patients with myasthenia gravis are extremely sensitive to depolarizing neuromuscular blocking agents.

III.56   Prolonged neuromuscular blockade is associated with:

1   Hyponatraemia.

2   Aminoglycosides.

3   Respiratory failure.

4   Pregnancy.

5   Angiotensin-converting enzyme (ACE) inhibitors.

III.57   Regarding shivering:

1   It occurs in 50% of cases.

2   It is independent of gender.

3   Opioids make shivering worse.

4   It is more likely if anticholinergic agents are used preoperatively.

5   It can be treated with doxapram 0.2 mg kg^{-1}.

III.58   Concerning non-surgical complications of operations:

1   Corneal abrasions can be prevented by taping the eyes closed.

2   The incidence of post-intubation sore throats is 30%.

3   Brachial plexus damage is likely if the arm is adducted more than 90°.

4   The lithotomy position is associated with saphenous nerve damage.

5   The occiput is one of the three common sites of skin pressure damage in elderly surgical patients.

III.59   The indications for supporting ventilation in head-injured patients include:

1   A Glasgow Coma Scale (GCS) score of less than 10.

2   A PaO$_2$ of less than 9 kPa on air.

3 Hyperventilation – a respiratory rate greater then 20.
4 Hypotension.
5 Seizure activity.

III.60 Concerning the management of a fractured maxilla:

1 Maxillary fractures are usually isolated injuries.
2 Closed head injuries and maxillary fractures are an indication for tracheostomy.
3 Nasal tubes should only be used with awake fibre-optic intubation techniques.
4 Oral intubation is usually straightforward.
5 Blood loss is rarely severe.

III.61 The following are of proven value in the treatment of pulmonary contusion:

1 Prophylactic antibiotics.
2 Continuous positive-airways pressure (CPAP).
3 Colloid infusion.
4 Encouragement of a profound diuresis.
5 Steroids.

III.62 The following conditions may predispose to the development of adult respiratory distress syndrome (ARDS):

1 Severe intra-abdominal sepsis.
2 Prolonged therapy with a high concentration of oxygen.
3 Burns to the trunk and limbs.
4 Renal failure.
5 Haemorrhagic shock.

III.63 Concerning gut motility:

1 Cisapride is ineffective if atropine is co-administered.
2 Oculogyric crises can occur with metoclopramide.
3 Erythromycin causes diarrhoea.
4 Erythromycin should be given in reduced doses in hepatic failure.
5 Cisapride prolongs the prothrombin time in patients on warfarin.

III.64 Concerning indirect calorimetry:

1 It measures the rate of oxidation of metabolic substrates.
2 It uses the volume of oxygen consumed.

3 It estimates the volume of carbon dioxide produced.
4 Both inspired and expired minute volumes must be measured.
5 The energy expended is calculated with the de Weir formula.

III.65 Concerning malaria:

1 Hyponatraemia is common.
2 Patients with *Plasmodium falciparum* have paroxysms of fever.
3 Cerebral malaria causes seizures.
4 Leucocytosis is a feature of malaria.
5 An exchange transfusion may be necessary if the patient is severely ill.

III.66 With regard to multiple trauma:

1 Hypothermia frequently masks hypovolaemia.
2 Tissue oxygen debt does not lead to late-onset organ dysfunction.
3 A haemoglobin of 8 g dl^{-1} is an acceptable level for oxygen delivery.
4 Rhabdomyolysis may occur following limb injuries.
5 Prophylactic antibiotics are of limited use.

III.67 Concerning overdosage with amphetamine or related compounds:

1 It may lead to hallucinations.
2 It increases central dopamine release.
3 Hypothermia is a common complication.
4 Muscle rigidity if present responds to dantrolene.
5 Water intoxication is common after amphetamine overdosage.

III.68 Regarding botulism:

1 It is rarely lethal.
2 It is a food-borne disease.
3 It can cause parasympathetic symptoms.
4 Late-onset cases are usually more seriously ill.
5 Magnesium protects against the effect of the toxin.

III.69 The following are common nephrotoxins:

1 Phenytoin.
2 Propofol.
3 Radiographic contrast.

4   Narcotics.

5   Herbal medicines.

III.70   The following are recognized features of a pulmonary embolism:

1   Pleuritic chest pain.

2   A normal chest X-ray.

3   Preference for sitting upright.

4   ECG signs of left ventricular strain.

5   Raised levels of D-dimers.

III.71   Aprotinin:

1   Is a synthetic specific protease inhibitor.

2   Effects are concentration dependent.

3   Causes kallikrein inhibition.

4   Has a half-life of 4 hours.

5   Prevents inappropriate platelet activation by cathepsin G.

III.72   The following are used as neuroprotective agents:

1   Frusemide.

2   Nimodepine.

3   Dexamethasone.

4   Midazolam.

5   Morphine.

III.73   Near-infrared spectroscopy:

1   Uses light in the 1000–1200 mm wavelength.

2   Measures cytochrome aa3 concentrations.

3   Measures myoglobin.

4   Correlates with the xenon method of calculating cerebral blood flow.

5   Is stable during patient motion.

III.74   Concerning pressure sores in ICU:

1   Poor skin integrity is a major risk for pressure sores.

2   An air mattress is occasionally necessary for patients with burns.

3   An air mattress should replace the standard mattress.

4   An air loss bed reduces the contact pressure below capillary occlusion pressure.

5   An air fluidized bed allows manipulation of the patient's temperature.

III.75 Regarding peritoneal dialysis:

1 It is labour intensive.
2 It uses a sterile solution containing potassium.
3 Glucose is rarely added because of the slow exchange time.
4 Fluid leakage is a problem in the elderly.
5 Heparin 500 IU l^{-1} is usually added to the solutions used to prevent clotting.

III.76 Continuous positive-airways pressure (CPAP):

1 Can cause an increase in $PaCO_2$.
2 Raises intracranial pressure.
3 Improves left heart failure.
4 Rarely causes gastric dilation.
5 Has no effect on venous return.

III.77 With regard to hepatic encephalopathy:

1 Grade 2 equates to a confused patient with an altered mood.
2 Grade 3 equates to a stuporose patient, who may also be very confused and agitated.
3 The risk of cerebral oedema is over 50% in patients with Grade 3 encephalopathy.
4 Bradycardia is an early sign of cerebral oedema.
5 A head-up position is helpful.

III.78 Regarding meningitis:

1 *Listeria monocytogenes* causes seizures and focal lesions.
2 The diagnosis of bacterial meningitis is by culture of the cerebrospinal fluid (CSF).
3 A normal computed tomography (CT) scan excludes a raised intracranial pressure in these patients.
4 Dexamethasone should be given.
5 Signs in the elderly are unchanged from those seen in younger patients.

III.79 Hypomagnesaemia:

1 Leads to coma.
2 Seizures are unlikely.
3 May be caused by severe diarrhoea.
4 Is symptomatic below a plasma level of 0.5 mmol l^{-1}.
5 Occurs in alcoholics.

III.80 The effects of near-drowning in fresh water include:

1 Loss of alveolar surfactant.
2 Marked haemodynamic instability.
3 Hypothermia.
4 Mild metabolic acidosis.
5 Pulmonary oedema.

III.81 Lower oesophageal sphincter tone is increased by:

1 Metoclopramide.
2 Atropine.
3 Neostigmine.
4 Glucagon.
5 Gastric inhibitory peptide.

III.82 The following physical methods are used in anaesthesia to measure gaseous carbon dioxide concentrations:

1 Absorption spectroscopy.
2 Polarography.
3 Refractometry.
4 Solubility methods.
5 Paramagnetic analysis.

III.83 Regarding Class I medical equipment:

1 It has double insulation.
2 A fuse is incorporated into the circuit.
3 It is internally powered.
4 It has a connection between any conducting part (available to the operator) and earth.
5 The fuse rating, in amps, indicates the value at which it will 'blow'.

III.84 Concerning pressure transducers:

1 The first harmonic in Fourier analysis of an arterial pressure is the same as the pulse rate.
2 The third Fourier harmonic is three times the pulse rate.
3 Fourier analysis is phase independent in most clinical situations.
4 Damping has minimal effect on phase shifts.
5 The measuring system (transducer, catheter and tubing) should have a resonant frequency of approximately 20 Hz.

III.85 The following are true:

1 99.7% of observations will fall within 6 standard deviations of the mean.
2 95% of observations will fall within 1.96 standard deviations of the mean.
3 The chance of the next observation in a series falling outside the 95th confidence range is 5%.
4 A type 1 error is when the null hypothesis is falsely accepted.
5 The Mann–Whitney test is suitable only for parametric data.

III.86 The following are true in the context of electrical safety:

1 An earth leakage circuit breaker will protect patients from a short circuit across the live and neutral poles.
2 CF is the appropriate standard for equipment used for direct cardiac monitoring.
3 Surgical diathermy uses frequencies in the megahertz range.
4 The charge potential of the capacitor in an external defibrillator is of the order of 2000 V.
5 The average transthoracic impedance is 70–80 Ω.

III.87 The following are correct concerning the colligative properties of a solution when more solute is added to the solvent:

1 The vapour pressure is lowered.
2 The boiling point is depressed.
3 The osmotic pressure is increased.
4 The freezing point is depressed.
5 The colligative properties are described by Renault's law.

III.88 Scavenging and pollution in anaesthesia:

1 Many volatile anaesthetic agents affect the fertility of female theatre workers.
2 The maximum recommended level of nitrous oxide in the working environment is 100 ppm.
3 The maximum recommended level of isoflurane is greater in the UK than in the USA.
4 Passive scavenging systems are adversely affected by external factors such as wind conditions.
5 The UK standard is given in BS 6834.

III.89 The following relate to the measurement of cardiac output:

1 The Fick principle is based on the conservation of mass.
2 Thermodilution methods use a modified Stewart–Hamilton equation.

3 Continuous thermodilution methods use small surges of heat, of the order of 0.5°C.

4 Continuous thermodilution measurement is calculated and displayed in real time.

5 Doppler calculations depend on an accurate measurement of the cross-sectional area of the aorta.

III.90 **Considering the use of lasers:**

1 Characteristics of coherent radiation include collimation.

2 Lasers are monochromic.

3 Coherence is where all waves of light are parallel.

4 Vaporized tissue smoke, the 'laser plume', is sterile.

5 Class 2 lasers are low power and will not damage the eye in normal use.

III.1 Causes of secondary hyperparathyroidism include:

1 True   2 True   3 True   4 False   5 False

III.2 Regarding multiple endocrine neoplasia type 1 (MEN 1):

1 False   2 True   3 False   4 False   5 True

III.3 The following cause a raised serum creatine kinase concentration:

1 True   2 True   3 False   4 True   5 True

III.4 Phenoxybenzamine:

1 False   2 False   3 True   4 True   5 False

III.5 The following may result in massive haemoptysis:

1 True   2 True   3 True   4 True   5 True

III.6 Wegener's granulomatosis:

1 True   2 False   3 True   4 True   5 False

III.7 The following regarding inherited disorders of haemostasis are true:

1 False   2 False   3 False   4 True   5 False

III.8 With regard to familial periodic paralysis:

1 False   2 True   3 True   4 True   5 True

It is an autosomal dominant condition with variable penetrance.

III.9 Concerning renal function:

1 False   2 True   3 False   4 False   5 True

III.10 Subarachnoid haemorrhage:

1 False   2 False   3 False   4 False   5 True

III.11 Regarding atrial fibrillation and its treatment:

1 True   2 True   3 False   4 False   5 False

III.12 The following clinical conditions produce a right-to-left shunt:

1 True   2 False   3 True   4 False   5 False

A pulmonary embolism increases alveolar dead space. Fallot's tetralogy includes a ventricular septal defect coupled with right ventricular outflow tract obstruction, causing blood to shunt from right to left. Coarctation of the aorta is usually post-ductal and produces no shunt. Patent ductus arteriosus produces a left-to-right shunt.

III.13 Haemoglobin A:

1 True   2 True   3 True   4 True   5 False

2,3-DPG reduces the affinity of haemoglobin for oxygen, shifting the oxyhaemoglobin dissociation curve to the right. Fetal haemoglobin has less affinity for 2,3-DPG than haemoglobin A, thus promoting oxygen transfer from mother to fetus. The iron atom of the haem molecule remains in the ferrous state in the formation of oxyhaemoglobin. Oxidation of iron to the ferric state forms methaemoglobin.

III.14 The administration of magnesium may result in:

1 False   2 True   3 True   4 False   5 True

Magnesium exerts a presynaptic effect limiting acetylcholine release, resulting in a degree of neuromuscular block. The resulting decrease in mechanical ventilatory power may cause a decrease in FVC. Other effects include a prolongation of Q–T interval and bronchodilation.

III.15 A long Q–T interval may occur with:

1 True   2 False   3 True   4 True   5 False

Hypocalcaemia causes a prolonged Q–T interval. Digoxin has the opposite effect.

III.16	von Willebrand's disease:

1 True	2 False	3 True	4 False	5 False

Deficiency of von Willebrand factor causes a decrease in platelet adhesiveness, deficiency of factor VIII and abnormal vascular endothelium. The features are thus those of poor platelet function, with epistaxis and ecchymosis rather than haemarthrosis and haematomata. The bleeding time is prolonged but the prothrombin time is normal. Desmopressin is used to increase levels of factor VIII and von Willebrand factor. Platelet function may thus improve but their quantity is unchanged.

III.17	Features of hypothyroidism include:

1 True	2 True	3 False	4 True	5 True

In hypothyroidism there may be a brisk ankle jerk followed by delayed relaxation of the muscles.

III.18	Regarding epiglottitis:

1 False	2 True	3 False	4 False	5 True

III.19	The following changes may be seen in animals after hepatectomy:

1 False. The liver is the main site of glycogen storage which leads to hyperglycaemia when storage cannot occur.

2 False. The liver is the only site of albumin formation; a fall in the ratio is inevitable but will be slow because of the long half-life of albumin in the circulation.

3 True. There is a decreased incorporation of non-esterified fatty acids into triglycerides and lipoproteins.

4 False. This process occurs in the lungs.

5 True

III.20	Parathyroid hormone secretion increases in response to:

1 False	2 False	3 False	4 False	5 True

III.21	The following are consistent with a diagnosis of neuroleptic malignant syndrome:

| 1 True | 2 False | 3 False | 4 False | 5 False |

III.22	Dexmedetomidine:

| 1 False | 2 False | 3 False | 4 False | 5 False |

III.23	The following are associated with an increased risk of perioperative peripheral neuropathy of the corresponding nerves:

| 1 False | 2 True | 3 False | 4 True | 5 False |

III.24	With regard to the oculocardiac reflex (OCR):

| 1 False | 2 True | 3 False | 4 False | 5 True |

The oculocardiac reflex consists of faintness, nausea and bradycardia, and may lead to asystolic cardiac arrest; it commonly occurs due to stretching of the extraocular muscles. Retrobulbar anaesthesia does block the afferent limb of the reflex, while atropine blocks the efferent limb. There is an association between the oculocardiac reflex and postoperative vomiting.

III.25	The following are true of the hypoglossal nerve (CrXII):

| 1 True | 2 False | 3 True | 4 False | 5 True |

The hypoglossal nerve supplies motor function to all muscles of the tongue with the exception of palatoglossus. Its nucleus is in the floor of the fourth ventricle and it exits, like many of the lower cranial nerves, as a series of 'rootlets'. These combine to form the nerve before leaving through the hypoglossal canal. It lies between the carotid and internal jugular vain until about the angle of the mandible, when it loops around the lingual artery, on its way to directly supply the muscles of the tongue. It also has a descending branch that joins that fibres from C1, C2 and C3 to supply the muscles supporting the hyoid bone: sternohyoid, omohyoid and geniohyoid.

III.26	Ropivacaine:

| 1 False | 2 False | 3 False | 4 True | 5 False |

III.27	Regarding postherpetic neuralgia:

| 1 False | 2 False | 3 False | 4 False | 5 True |

III.28	Physiological dead space:

| 1 True | 2 False | 3 True | 4 False | 5 True |

Physiological dead space changes with tidal volume. It can be calculated using the Bohr equation:

$$\frac{V_D}{V_T} = \frac{PaCO_2 - PeCO_2}{PaCO_2}$$

In the normal subject, the PCO_2 in alveolar gas and arterial blood are virtually identical and $PaCO_2$ can be used.

III.29	A 3.1 kg baby delivered at 39 weeks' gestation presents with respiratory distress due to a congenital diaphragmatic hernia 6 hours after birth:

| 1 False | 2 True | 3 False | 4 False | 5 False |

Current practice favours stabilization of the baby prior to surgery. The prerequisites are a normal acid–base balance, effective gas exchange and control of any persisting fetal circulation. Induction of anaesthesia prior to intubation carries the risk of forcing gas into the stomach by face mask intermittent positive-pressure ventilation and further compromising ventilation. The room temperature needs to be about 30°C when the baby is exposed for induction and placing of the monitoring, but can safely be reduced for surgery to enable comfortable conditions for the operating department staff. The haematocrit at birth is normally 52–58%. Arterial oxygen saturation of above 95% places the baby at risk from retrolental fibroplasias.

III.30	The following drugs are reduced by plasma cholinesterase (pseudocholinestrase):

| 1 False | 2 False | 3 False | 4 False | 5 False |

Plasma cholinesterase hydrolyses (it does not reduce) mivacurium, suxamethonium and amethocaine. Remifentanil is metabolized by non-specific plasma and tissue esterases.

III.31	Functional residual capacity is increased by:

| 1 False | 2 True | 3 True | 4 True | 5 True |

functional residual capacity (FRC) is the volume of lung remaining after expiration during tidal ventilation. Oxygen replaces nitrogen in the FRC during pre-oxygenation but the volume does not increase. PEEP and CPAP exert their clinical action by increasing FRC. Increased airway resistance increases FRC.

III.32	**The IUPAC nomenclature of hydrocarbons:**
	1 False 2 True 3 True 4 True 5 False

The International Union of Pure and Applied Chemistry method is precise, but is only one of several systems of nomenclature. The longest unbranched chain is named as the last part of the description (the number of bonds determines what it is: single bonds are alkanes, double are alkenes and triple bonds are alkynes). Examples would include 3,4-dimethylheptane.

III.33	**The cell cycle of a eukaryotic cell includes the following phases:**
	1 True 2 True 3 False 4 True 5 False

The cycle starts with G_0 and passes through G_1 with cell growth and normal metabolic activity. Phase S is that of DNA replication leading to preparation for cell division – G_2, and ending with cell division – mitosis or meiosis – phase M.

III.24	**The following are true in patients with untreated hypertension:**
	1 False 2 True 3 False 4 True 5 True

The British Hypertension Society recommends treatment of sustained systolic pressures above 200 mmHg or diastolic pressures above 110 mmHg. Only 10% of patients have an identifiable cause such as renal or endocrine disease, pregnancy, coarctation of the aorta or taking the oral contraceptive pill. Malignant hypertension still requires urgent treatment in hospital, usually by oral drug therapy.

III.35	**The following changes occur in the nervous system with ageing alone:**
	1 False 2 True 3 True 4 False 5 True

There is a generalized loss of cells, synapses and neurotransmitters with ageing. This affects all neurological systems including the autonomic system, for instance, leading to postural hypotension. The loss of myelin leads to delayed motor conduction and increasing immobility and instability. Deafness affects up to 36% of all people over 70 years.

III.36 In Hirschsprung's disease:

1 False 2 True 3 True 4 True 5 False

The primary site is colonic. There is a strong association between central alveolar hypoventilation (Ondine's curse) and Hirschsprung's disease. The poor muscular coordination of the gut predisposes to vomiting. It is more common in males, and has a multifactorial inheritance (it used to be thought to be an autosomal recessive trait).

III.37 Halothane hepatitis:

1 True 2 True 3 True 4 False 5 False

There have only been a handful of proven cases (7) of halothane hepatic necrosis, but there are far more common disturbances in liver function. Type 1 dysfunction is limited to a rise in enzymes up to three times normal that occurs within 2 weeks of exposure. The very rare Type 2 (1:37 000) massive hepatic necrosis is an oxidative process, although it was originally believed to be a reductive process. It is a specific trifluoroacetyl oxidative metabolite that is believed to be the cause (this is not produced by the metabolism of sevoflurane).

III.38 Etomidate:

1 True 2 False 3 False 4 False 5 True

It is prepared in 35% propylene glycol and has a pH of 8.1. It causes very little histamine release and has an incidence of hypersensitivity of between 1:50 000 to 1:450 000.

III.39 Active transport across a cell membrane:

1 False 2 True 3 True 4 False 5 True

The difference between facilitated diffusion and active transport is the ability to work against a concentration gradient and gradients of 30:1 for potassium have been identified. Sugars are actively transported in the gut and kidney, but use facilitated diffusion everywhere else.

III.40 Regarding sterilization:

1 True 2 False 3 False 4 False 5 True

Autoclaving is a function of time, pressure of the steam and its temperature. Dry heat is used for glass equipment, but there has to be a gradual change in temperature to prevent too rapid expansion and breakage. Gamma radiation equipment is too expensive for hospital use, and is limited to industrial pre-packaged items. The American Centers for Disease Control and Prevention define three categories of risk: critical, semi-critical and non-critical. The first relates to any equipment that enters a patient's body through the skin or a mucous membrane; semi-critical ones are in contact but do not penetrate the patient. Face masks are included in this category, but are often treated as non-critical, and disinfection is a reasonable and acceptable method of cleaning.

III.41	The clotting factors' common names are as follows:
	1 True　2 False　3 True　4 False　5 True

Factor VI is unused in respect of the commonly used terms. Factor V is proaccelerin, accelerator globulin or prothrombokinase and factor X is the Stuart–Prower or Stuart factor.

III.42	Concerning suxamethonium apnoea:
	1 False　2 False　3 True　4 False　5 False

Diamorphine, mivacurium, procaine and cocaine are all metabolized by plasma cholinesterase. While DNA analysis is the most accurate method of identifying abnormalities, it has not replaced the simpler dibucaine/fluoride screening. The use of fresh frozen plasma cannot be recommended because the effective concentration of plasma cholinesterase in the donated units is unknown, there is always a compatibility and infective risk with blood product use, and this should be a benign, self-limiting and safely managed complication. Succinyl monocholine has about 1:20 of the activity of the parent compound.

III.43	Concerning gross obesity:
	1 False　2 False　3 False　4 True　5 True

The standard table will support 24 stone. Gas exchange is impaired because of a reduced lung capacity, increased closing volume and a decreased functional residual capacity, leading to a fall in oxygen tension of up to 20%. Arterial PCO_2 is usually normal. Polycythaemia indicates daytime hypoxia and is an ominous sign of respiratory failure in these patients. The inaccuracy of non-invasive blood pressure recording and the prolonged nature of all but the most minor of procedures suggest that an arterial line is inserted. This is often less technically demanding than finding reasonable venous access. The risks of aspiration and loss of the airway on induction are so great that awake intubation should always be considered in the grossly obese.

III.44 Considering regional anaesthesia in the near-term obstetric patient:

1 False   2 False   3 False   4 True   5 False

Ephedrine reduced fetal cord pH more than phenylephrine. Aortocaval compression is more of a problem because there is already a reduced circulating blood volume – lower limb flow decreases and upper limb vasoconstriction occurs as a compensatory process. The epidural venous congestion is a less likely reason than altered neuronal sensitivity possibly induced by progesterone. The signs of blood loss (changes in heart rate and blood pressure) remain and, although there may be less blood loss under regional anaesthesia, the volume lost may be great and rapid and replacement must be appropriate.

III.45 With regard to opioid receptors:

1 True   2 False   3 False   4 True   5 True

The recent classification is into OP1 (delta), OP2 (kappa), OP3 (mu) and ORL1 (orphan) receptors. Currently no subtypes are believed to exist for the opioid receptors. The postsynaptic receptors are linked to potassium channels and, when stimulated, enhance potassium outflow as well as stabilizing the membrane.

III.46 Considering a patient with jaundice:

1 False   2 False   3 True   4 True   5 True

Clinical assessment will only correctly diagnose 65% of patients with jaundice, whereas biochemical and other investigations can increase this to 95%. The abnormal liver function tests indicate a 'spill-over' of intracellular contents rather than a reduction in the normal hepatic synthetic functions. Gilbert's syndrome – affecting about 5% of the population – leads to intermittent jaundice from unconjugated bilirubin.

III.47 Concerning adhesion molecules:

1 True   2 True   3 False   4 True   5 False

There is little direct anaesthetic research into adhesion molecules, but both halothane and sevoflurane alter expression of adhesion molecules. Integrins mediate cell-to-cell and cell-to-matrix expression. The other major group of adhesion molecules is the immunoglobulin superfamily.

III.48 Regarding arterial tourniquets:

> 1 False   2 True   3 True   4 True   5 False

Sickle disease states and peripheral vascular disease are absolute contraindications. The inflation times should be as short as possible, and if there is a surgical need for longer times, deflation and reinflation should occur frequently. The longer the duration of occlusion the greater the ischaemic load, and in frail patients the metabolic acidosis may cause hypotension. The cuff pressure should be titrated to the patient's systolic blood pressure and a pressure of 50 mmHg above systolic used.

III.49 Regarding Apert's syndrome:

> 1 True   2 True   3 False   4 True   5 False

The majority of cases arise sporadically, but it is a multi-system disorder caused by mutations of the fibroblast growth factor receptor-2 gene. There is a 10% incidence of cardiac defects, of which pulmonary stenosis, ventricular septal defects and an overriding aorta are the commonest. Cervical abnormalities leading to an unstable neck may complicate the compromised upper airway and should be actively sought. The scout film of the computed tomography series may be adequate, or a formal cervical film may be requested. Craniosynostosis is associated with a raised intracranial pressure and excessive premedication or hypoventilation should be avoided.

III.50 With regard to intracranial aneurysms:

> 1 True   2 False   3 True   4 True   5 False

The commonest site is the internal carotid system (41%), followed by the anterior cerebral artery (34%). Cerebral vasospasm occurs in 70% of patients, but is only symptomatic in about 20–30%. The peak incidence of vasospasm is at 7 days after the bleed.

III.51 Regarding dexamethasone and postoperative nausea and vomiting:

> 1 False   2 False   3 True   4 True   5 True

Dexamethasone has a slow onset of action, taking up to 2 hours to become effective, although it will then continue to provide anti-emetic cover for up to 24 hours. The optimal dosage has not been described, but most published data is with a dose of 8 mg, although 2.5 mg has been used with effect. It does reduce opiate-induced nausea and vomiting both in absolute frequency and in the severity of vomiting.

III.52   Concerning the basic mechanisms of anaesthesia:

| 1 True | 2 True | 3 False | 4 False | 5 True |

One argument for more specific sites of action of anaesthetic drugs is the finding that, in common with some non-anaesthetic drugs, learning can be suppressed. Most general anaesthetic vapours act on the $GABA_a$ receptor, but xenon and cyclopentone do not. The ion channels have not been defined directly; some inferences about their structure can be made by cryoelecton microscopy. The anaesthetic sites on excitable proteins are usually found on membrane proteins.

III.53   Concerning Parkinson's disease and anaesthesia:

| 1 True | 2 False | 3 False | 4 False | 5 True |

Over 80% of dopaminergic neurones have to be lost to cause symptoms. The disease is truly multi-systemic and affects all major areas of anaesthetic concern including respiratory, cardiovascular and neurological systems. Autonomic dysfunction is common, increasing the risk of aspiration, sleep apnoea, orthostatic hypotension and sialorrhoea.

III.54   Concerning neuropathic pain:

| 1 False | 2 True | 3 False | 4 True | 5 False |

Many examples of neuropathic pain do have an identifiable lesion, but others have no such cause. Allodynia also occurs in sunburn, for instance! While there are novel modalities for treatment in the pipeline, some have proved disappointing and a large multi-centre trial has not demonstrated any effect on the progression of diabetic neuropathy.

III.55   Concerning myasthenia gravis:

| 1 False | 2 True | 3 False | 4 True | 5 False |

Seventy-five per cent of patients have thymic dysfunction, of whom 85% have hyperplasia. The incidence is 1 in 10 000 of the population. They are unpredictably resistant to depolarizing and exquisitely sensitive to non-depolarizing neuromuscular blocking agents.

III.56   Prolonged neuromuscular blockade is associated with:

| 1 True | 2 True | 3 True | 4 False | 5 False |

Any metabolic disorder has the potential to prolong neuromuscular blockade, but low serum sodium, potassium or calcium and raised magnesium levels are common causes. Respiratory failure predisposes the patient to respiratory acidosis, which is a cause for prolongation of blockage. Normal pregnancy does not have an effect, nor do angiotensin-converting enzyme inhibitors.

III.57	Shivering:
	1 False 2 False 3 False 4 True 5 True

Shivering occurs in up to 65% of cases and is related to age and gender. Prolonged operations and anaesthetic technique are also important causes of hypothermia leading to shivering. Treatment can be with opioids or doxapram. Pethidine is suggested as being the most effective opioid in the recovery period. Clonidine is thought to prevent shivering if given on induction. The most effective treatment is to avoid hypothermia, for instance by using forced air mattresses. Treatment may need to start prior to induction of anaesthesia, especially in frail elderly patients.

III.58	Concerning non-surgical complications of operations:
	1 True 2 False 3 True 4 True 5 True

Post-intubation soreness is nearer to 50%, but may also be due to laryngoscopy, dry gases or laryngeal mask insertion. The lithotomy position can lead to pressure damage to either the common peroneal or saphenous nerves. Any dependent area can develop pressure damage if the underlying mattress or sheet is creased, but the occiput, elbows and heels are the most commonly affected areas.

III.59	The indications for supporting ventilation in head-injured patients include:
	1 False 2 True 3 False 4 False 5 False

A Glasgow Coma Scale score of 8 or less is the usual guideline for intubation and ventilation. Hyperventilation can only be accurately described in terms of end-tidal or preferably arterial CO_2 tension, and under 3.5 kPa is the figure used. Hypotension has no direct indication, but must be investigated further to identify and treat the cause. Fitting again is not a direct indication for intubation and ventilation unless the patient is to be transferred to a tertiary neurosurgical unit.

III.60	Concerning the management of a fractured maxilla:
	1 False 2 True 3 False 4 True 5 False

Maxillary fractures have to be assumed to be the result of severe trauma and will often be associated with head and neck injuries. Where these are present the expectation of a compromised airway makes the consideration of an early tracheostomy important. Surgical management usually involves plating and fixation without the need for the wiring or halo splints that previously were used. Arch bars to facilitate rubber band fixation may be placed if there appears to be an unsatisfactory alignment after reduction and stabilization. The nasal route should not be used because of the high risk of a basal skull fracture. Blood loss from damage to the maxillary artery can be severe and should be predicted and suitable precautions taken.

III.61　The following are of proven value in the treatment of pulmonary contusion:

　1 False　　2 True　　3 False　　4 False　　5 False

Prophylactic antibiotics are of unproven benefit. CPAP is extremely helpful and may prevent the need for further ventilatory support. Neither colloidal infusion nor diuresis is of benefit. Steroids have no proven value and may increase the risk of sepsis.

III.62　The following conditions may predispose to the development of adult respiratory distress syndrome (ARDS):

　1 True　　2 True　　3 True　　4 False　　5 True

Uncomplicated renal failure has no direct association with ARDS.

III.63　Concerning gut motility:

　1 True　　2 True　　3 False　　4 True　　5 True

Gut motility is increased to treat patients with ileus, vomiting or who have large gastric aspirates. Erythromycin is a motilin agonist and causes few side effects.

III.64　Concerning indirect calorimetry:

　1 True　　2 True　　3 False　　4 False　　5 True

Both oxygen and carbon dioxide volumes are measured. However, 1-minute volume can be calculated if the other is measured, and the oxygen and carbon dioxide concentrations are also known. The Haldane transformation is used:

$$Vi = Ve \times \frac{Ne}{Ni}$$

The de Weir formula is:

Energy expenditure $= (3.94\,VO_2 + 1.11\,VCO_2) \times 1.44$

III.65	Concerning malaria:
	1 True 2 False 3 True 4 False 5 True

P. falciparum is rarely associated with a classical fever pattern of alternating swings in feeling hot/cold. Equally a leucocytosis is unusual in malaria. The greater the percentage of parasitaemia the more severe the features of the disease and if greater than 10% (or if the patient is severely ill) exchange transfusion of 2–3 litres may be necessary.

III.66	With regard to multiple trauma:
	1 True 2 False 3 False 4 True 5 False

Even up to 7 days after the injury, multiple organ dysfunction can occur because of a persisting tissue oxygen debt. Early and complete resuscitation should be achieved. The balance of evidence suggests a level of 9–10 g dl^{-1} is important, and should be maintained by transfusion where needed. Prophylactic antibiotics may need to be given for a couple of weeks and do have a beneficial effect.

III.67	Concerning overdosage with amphetamine or related compounds:
	1 True 2 True 3 False 4 True 5 False

High doses lead to central nervous system hyperactivity. Hyperthermia, agitation and seizures may occur, and may progress to coma or liver failure. Water intoxication is usually seen in 'ecstasy' or 'eve' ingestion in hot nightclubs.

III.68	Regarding botulism:
	1 False 2 True 3 True 4 False 5 False

Botulism is still a very lethal disease and the faster the onset the more dangerous it is. Magnesium exacerbates the effects of the toxin and products containing it should be avoided. If the patient survives, resolution is slow over a period of several weeks.

III.69   The following are common nephrotoxins:

1 True   2 False   3 True   4 False   5 True

III.70   The following are recognized features of a pulmonary embolism:

1 True   2 True   3 False   4 False   5 True

The patient with an acute pulmonary embolism prefers to lie flat, and has right ventricular strain.

III.71   Aprotinin:

1 False   2 True   3 True   4 False   5 True

Aprotinin is a non-specific naturally occurring serum protease inhibitor and at low concentration it inhibits fibrinolysis and complement activation. At higher ones it inhibits kallikrein. It has a half-life of 3 hours.

III.72   The following are used as neuroprotective agents:

1 True   2 True   3 True   4 False   5 False

The mechanisms involved are usually attempts to reduce cerebral oedema or vasospasm or to decrease the cerebral metabolic rate. They are usually used against a background of generalized sedation.

III.73   Near-infrared spectroscopy:

1 False   2 True   3 True   4 True   5 False

It uses near-infrared (700–1000 mm) light, and also measures oxy- and deoxyhaemoglobin as well as myoglobin. It is very sensitive to motion artefact because photon capture devices have to be used to sense the transmitter light. They may be sensitive to high levels of ambient light for the same reason.

III.74   Concerning pressure sores in ITU:

1 True   2 False   3 False   4 False   5 True

Air mattresses are the minimum requirement for any patient with poor skin integrity and can replace or lie on top of the standard mattress. The air fluidized bed is the only one to reduce the contact pressure and also allows control of the ambient temperature.

III.75	Regarding peritoneal dialysis:
1 True	2 False	3 False	4 True	5 False

Glucose is used to alter the tonicity of the solution and potassium is not used because it is so slowly equilibrated through the peritoneum. Heparin may be used for the first few cycles (up to six) but not thereafter.

III.76	Continuous positive-airways pressure (CPAP):
1 True	2 True	3 True	4 False	5 False

CPAP raises intrathoracic pressure and can lead to air trapping. Even low pressures can lead to gastric dilation and an increased risk of aspiration. Modern nasal and face masks are much more comfortable and are well tolerated by the majority of patients.

III.77	With regard to hepatic encephalopathy:
1 False	2 True	3 True	4 False	5 True

The highest grade is 4, which is comatose. The higher the grade, the more likely is cerebral oedema, which is the commonest cause of death. Intracranial pressure (ICP) monitoring should be considered and the late signs of bradycardia, hypertension and muscle rigidity are very serious signs of a raised ICP.

III.78	Regarding meningitis:
1 True	2 False	3 False	4 True	5 False

The CT scan may not show signs of a raised intracranial pressure and lumbar puncture may still be dangerous. The diagnosis is made on examination of the CSF, the delay to achieve results from culture is too long to delay treatment in such a lethal condition and empirical therapy is necessary. The elderly may have very subtle changes and diagnosis may be very difficult.

III.79	Hypomagnesaemia:
1 False	2 False	3 True	4 True	5 True

Magnesium is an intracellular ion and the plasma levels are a poor reflection of the degree of deficit. Neuronal hyperactivity is caused and agitation, seizures and confusion are seen. Other signs are similar to low potassium or calcium, muscle weakness, lethargy or arrhythmias.

III.80 | The effects of near-drowning in fresh water include:

1 True   2 False   3 True   4 False   5 False

Twenty per cent of patients have acute laryngospasm with airway protection, but there does not appear to be a marked difference between fresh and sea water near-drowning. Most have a lung injury, hypothermia which can be profound, and the effects of an episode of prolonged hypoxia. Metabolic acidosis is usually severe and will require aggressive therapy.

III.81 | Lower oesophageal sphincter tone is increased by:

1 True   2 False   3 True   4 False   5 False

Lower oesophageal sphincter tone is partly maintained by vagal input. This explains the relaxing effects of atropine and neostigmine.

III.82 | The following physical methods are used in anaesthesia to measure gaseous carbon dioxide concentrations:

1 True   2 False   3 True   4 True   5 False

Polarography and paramagnetic analysis techniques are used to measure oxygen concentrations. Other methods of measuring carbon dioxide include Ramon scattering, mass spectrometry and photoacoustic measurements.

III.83 | Regarding Class I medical equipment:

1 False   2 True   3 False   4 True   5 False

Double insulation is a characteristic of Class II equipment and internal power of Class III. The fuse rating is the maximum current that the fuse will survive for 1000 hours. The majority of anaesthetic equipment is Class II and does not require earthing because of the double insulation or reinforced insulation. Class III equipment is usually portable and battery powered.

III.84	Concerning pressure transducers:

1 True	2 True	3 False	4 False	5 False

The harmonic components of a complex wave travel at different velocities along the tubing, and the fidelity of the system will be increasingly distorted the longer the tube is. Optimal damping (D = 0.64) slows down the speed of all harmonics and although the response time is reduced the fidelity is improved. The system has to have as high a resonant frequency as possible, usually about 100 Hz, and the manufacturers try to achieve a flat response over the clinical range of 10–30 Hz. The use of long, soft catheters will reduce the resonant frequency of the system towards the clinical range and reduce accuracy.

III.85	The following are true:

1 True	2 True	3 True	4 False	5 False

A type 1 error is where the null hypothesis falsely rejected; type 2 errors usually occur when the sample is too small to display that there is a real difference between the groups. By definition a type 1 error will occur 5% of the time if the level of significance has been defined as $p < 0.05$. The statistical tests used for non-parametric data can also be used for normally distributed data, although they are less precise than ones designed for normally distributed data.

III.86	The following are true in the context of electrical safety:

1 False	2 True	3 True	4 False	5 True

Earth leakage circuit breakers do not protect against direct short circuits. CF is the highest standard for leakage currents in monitoring equipment; the C stands for cardiac use, while the F denotes a floating (isolated) circuit. The charge capacitor in an external defibrillator is of the order of 4000–6000 V.

III.87	The following are correct concerning the colligative properties of a solution when more solute is added to the solvent:

1 True	2 False	3 True	4 True	5 False

The boiling point is increased because of the lower vapour pressure at a given temperature. It is Raoult's law that states that the depression of the freezing point is proportional to the molar concentration of the solute, as is the lowering of the vapour pressure.

III.88	Scavenging and pollution in anaesthesia:

1 False	2 True	3 True	4 True	5 True

There is no evidence that any anaesthetic vapour leads to infertility, spontaneous abortion, cancer, liver or kidney disease, or blood dyscrasias. Concerns about neurological symptoms and intellectual impairment are also unfounded. However, nitrous oxide does affect red cell maturation and has been reported to cause a polyneuropathy in exposed dental surgeons. Passive systems are vulnerable to atmospheric changes around the gas outlet, whereas active systems are less affected. BS 6834 (1987) remains the current standard.

III.89	The following relate to the measurement of cardiac output:

1 True	2 True	3 False	4 False	5 True

The continuous thermodilution systems calculate the cardiac output every 30–90 seconds, but average the data over about 10 minutes. This slow response remains a major limitation to its practical use in rapidly changing situations. Doppler-derived cardiac output depends on an accurate measurement of the aortic cross-sectional area, laminar flow of the blood in the aorta, both the measurement of the velocity and flow being made at the same site, and there being a parallel angle between the blood flow and the Doppler beam.

III.90	Considering the use of lasers:

1 True	2 True	3 False	4 False	5 True

Lasers are beams of coherent light that is monochromatic, parallel (collimated) and the waves are all in phase (coherent). Vaporized smoke can contain infective particles and can infect the respiratory tract or cause nausea. Class 2 lasers are of low power and the normal blink reflex will protect the eye.

The development of a short notes paper is based on the concept of covering a wider range of important topics than is possible in the traditional essay paper. Techniques that are suitable and successful for a detailed and logical description of a topic are often poor when time and conciseness are necessary. The benefit of multiple very short questions is that candidates have to demonstrate how they prioritize their knowledge and how they exercise their judgement.

There is no substitute for actually learning the core knowledge and of having given enough thought to the practice of anaesthesia, pain management and critical care.[1] However, even with this essential work completed, poor preparation and training in the skills for completing short notes may prove to be an insurmountable obstacle to success.

The Short Notes paper for the FRCA examination is a paper of 12 questions, all of which must be completed to achieve a pass (2) grade. If one question is missed the highest score is a fail (1+ that is possible to be redeemed) and the chances of success fall dramatically. The marking schedule allows for a margin of error within the total number of questions but each question is marked individually by two examiners on a pass, close fail or veto fail scheme. The aggregate mark then determines the outcome of the paper. Clearly it is better to have a solid basis of knowledge and be able to safely apply it than to be an expert in only a few areas.

The paper lasts for 3 hours and simple sums suggest that an allocation of no more than 15 minutes for each question is important. There has to be time to martial thoughts and rehearse the planned presentation of the answer. This not only allows a reflection on the appropriateness of the priority given, but also frequently suggests other aspects that must be mentioned. Time is vital, but an average of 3 minutes is the most commonly suggested time allocation. Write on the answer sheet and then cross it out. These musings are not marked or even scrutinized. There is no time (or marks) for a complete dissertation and the penalty of taking too long on one question is to guarantee doing another one badly.

There are several methods of determining in which order to answer the paper – do the ones you know most about first, or last. Do them in the printed order or choose the apparently simple ones first – anatomy, for instance, where a simple diagram may cover many aspects of the question. There really is no absolute guide, but common sense suggests that during the stress of the examination keeping to the order of the paper is the strategy least likely to result in missed questions. The penalty for doing this is far higher than answering the missed question poorly.

---

[1] As with the MCQ section, the content of these questions reflects elements of the curriculum of the final FRCA but they cannot be used in isolation or as a substitute for the comprehensive reading that is needed to acquire the depth of knowledge necessary for safe anaesthetic practice.

How should the questions be answered? By writing short notes! There is no time to waste on introductions, presentation of facts and then a discussion. Say what is of the utmost importance clearly and first – by single words or phrases if possible, then the second most critical and so on. If there could be doubt about your view of priority highlight or underline the phrase. Leave no possibility of misinterpretation by the two marking examiners. Remember that adding in second thoughts confirms poor judgement and must be avoided by effective use of the 3-minute preparatory time. If you do suddenly think of something, write it in a different coloured ink and review at the end of the paper (with the answers) if you were right to add it or not. Next time check for similar aspects in the initial 3 minutes.

Practice is essential. The papers presented here are from the ones published in *Current Anaesthesia and Critical Care* and were written by experts in these fields. That does not mean that there is only the one correct answer. The suggested answers give a guide to the importance and relevance of the facts and where they fall in a clinical sense; for instance, high science may not be more important than clinical, life-saving aspects.

The aim of using these papers is to develop a method of answering the questions in the time allowed, and also to lead to discussion about the aspects of the questions and answers that you disagree with. This practice, leading up to the final FRCA, is most effective if a group of colleagues can meet and sit the same paper at the same time, or arrange to sit it and then meet to review their own answers and the suggested ones. At this stage of preparation, being right is far less important than developing a sound strategy for answering the paper.

Some of these answers include some useful references for further reading.

Paper One Write short notes on the following topics. Do not miss out any questions and remember that there are only 3 hours in total to complete this paper.

1   Adverse reactions to anaesthesia
2   The two eye blocks commonly used for cataract surgery
3   Anaesthetic considerations for general surgery in heart/lung-transplanted patients
4   The sitting position for neurosurgery
5   Temperature control in theatre
6   Volume of distribution
7   Amiodarone
8   Extracorporeal membrane oxygenation in neonates
9   Lithium therapy and anaesthesia
10 The pathophysiology of drowning and the resuscitation of a victim of near-drowning
11 The transurethral resection of prostate (TURP) syndrome
12 The cleaning and sterilization of anaesthetic equipment

1 Adverse reactions to anaesthesia

Serious adverse reactions to anaesthesia are, fortunately, rare, an incidence of 1:900–1:20 000 being quoted in the literature. Many mechanisms are implicated. Those involving IgE or IgG are termed anaphylactic, those of a non-immune mechanism being termed anaphylactoid. Both release histamine from mast cells.

Whatever the mechanism, there are mediators released that cause hypotension, bronchospasm, pulmonary oedema, erythema, urticaria and swelling. The incidence seems to be increased in atopic individuals and shows a greater preponderance in women. While many anaesthetic drugs are implicated such as induction agents, analgesics and antibiotics, the neuromuscular junction blockers are amongst the most commonly implicated. Antibiotics, colloids, protamine and latex are also known to trigger adverse reactions.

Some indication of risk may be gleaned from the history or from the presence of atopy but frequently there will be no obvious predisposition.

In the event of the occurrence of such an adverse reaction one should summon help, stop the administration of any possible causative agent, give 100% oxygen and commence cardiopulmonary resuscitation if necessary. For cardiovascular collapse, adrenaline, α-agonists and fluids are indicated. For respiratory collapse, adrenaline, nebulized β_2 agonists and isoflurane should be considered. Intubation may be necessary either to maintain adequate oxygenation or to maintain the airway if angio-oedema is a problem.

Blood samples taken soon after the acute event should be analysed for mast cell tryptase, a protease found in mast cell granules. Levels will be increased following activation of mast cells. If levels are found to be raised then, following the patient's recovery, further investigation should be made. At about 4–6 weeks after the event, skin testing should be performed. If a true allergy is demonstrated then it is important that the patient carries a permanent reminder, such as a 'medic-alert' bracelet.

Further reading

Edwards IR, Aronson JK. Adverse drug reactions: definitions, diagnosis, and management. Uppsala Monitoring Centre, WHO Collaborating Centre for International Drug Monitoring, Sweden. *Lancet* 2000; 356(9237): 1255–1259

2 The two eye blocks commonly used for cataract surgery

The two local anaesthetic blocks commonly used for cataract surgery are retrobulbar blocks and peribulbar blocks. Both are suitable for procedures of up to around 1 hour duration, on cooperative patients with no coagulation disturbances or allergies to the local anaesthetic to be used (which is extremely rare). The presence of a chronic cough, the inability to lie still, the inability to lie flat, or a problem such as a facial tic are contraindications (although one could perform a facial nerve block in a patient with a chronic tic to attain immobility).

A retrobulbar block, where the local anaesthetic solution is injected behind the globe by passing the needle through the muscle cone, requires a smaller volume of local anaesthetic, as little as 2–3 ml of 2% lignocaine (usually with adrenaline). This block is of faster onset then a peribulbar block. In the peribulbar block, the local anaesthetic is injected around the globe, the muscle cone not being penetrated. This requires a greater volume of up to 10 ml of the aforementioned solution.

The injection of anaesthetic into the retrobulbar space may stimulate the oculocardiac reflex as the muscles are stretched. Other complications of a retrobulbar block include trauma to the vasculature, resulting in a retrobulbar haemorrhage (which can cause blindness owing to central retinal artery occlusion), injection into the cerebrospinal fluid, optic nerve damage and penetration of the globe. By contrast, the peribulbar approach, in which the cone of muscles is not penetrated, does not have the same incidence of these complications, as the anaesthetic is injected further from neural and vascular structures, but penetration of the globe is still possible.

As with all regional techniques it is essential that full facilities are immediately available for resuscitation.

Further reading

Troll GF. Regional ophthalmic anesthesia: safe techniques and avoidance of complications. *J Clin Anesth* 1995; 7(2): 163–172

Vaalamo MO, Paloheimo, Nikki PH. Painless needle insertion in regional anesthesia of the eye. *Anesth Analg* 1995; 80(4): 678–681

Wong DH. Regional anaesthesia for intraocular surgery. Wong DH. *Can J Anaesth* 1993; 40(7): 635–657

3 | **Anaesthetic considerations for general surgery in heart/lung transplanted patients**

General surgical conditions occurring in the early post-transplant period are usually related to the illness or the immune suppression drugs, e.g. pancreatitis or peptic ulceration. After the first month, surgical operations are required with the same frequency as in the non-transplanted population, although cholecystectomy may be more common secondary to cyclosporin use.

Physiologically, the heart has a higher resting rate of 100–120. Heart function is normal at rest. The Frank–Starling mechanism is normal, but the response to any increase in demand is slow. It responds poorly to sudden drops in preload. However, endogenous catecholamines will ensure that output will eventually equal demand. The respiratory problems may include a poor cough owing to recurrent laryngeal nerve and phrenic nerve palsies. Lung volumes are reduced, and a restrictive defect is common. Cachexia and renal dysfunction are common.

Any anaesthetic technique can be used but, although a regional technique may appear useful from the lung aspect, any drops in preload will be poorly tolerated cardiovascularly. Steroid cover will be required. Directly acting cardiovascular drugs such as adrenaline or isoprenaline should be ready. Cyclosporin prolongs and azathioprine shortens the duration of action of non-depolarizing neuromuscular blockers. A shortened endotracheal tube is necessary to avoid the tracheal anastomosis. Finally, it would seem advisable that even where the case has been entirely routine, postoperative care should be in a high-dependency or intensive care area.

4   The sitting position for neurosurgery

The advantages of the sitting position are ease of surgical access with good drainage and a good surgical field. The problems are associated with air embolism, pneumo-encephalus and postural hypotension. Generally, when a vein is cut during surgery it collapses, preventing an inflow of air; however, the venous sinuses are held open by the dura and entry of air can occur in up to 40% of patients. A large embolism entering the pulmonary bed will lead to a rise in pulmonary artery pressure, right ventricular strain, ventricular failure and a loss of cardiac output. The effect of ventilation–perfusion mismatch means the end-tidal carbon dioxide pressure will suddenly fall. Up to 25% of patients may have a patent foramen ovale, and with any increase of right atrial pressure air may be forced through and cause a paradoxical embolism.

Preventative and damage-limiting measures include avoidance of nitrous oxide, volume loading, positive end-expiratory pressure, controlled ventilation, anti-shock trousers and central venous catheters. Detection is aided by a high index of suspicion from the surgeon and the anaesthetist and the use of Doppler monitoring. The pulse oximeter, electrocardiograph and capnograph will all aid diagnosis and are routinely used. Upon detection, the position should be changed and the area flooded with saline; the inspired oxygen is increased to 100%. Attempts should be made to aspirate the air and to increase the venous pressure by jugular compression and intravenous fluids.

Further reading

Buhre W, Weyland A, Buhre K et al. Effects of the sitting position on the distribution of blood volume in patients undergoing neurosurgical procedures. *Br J Anaesth* 2000; 84(3): 354–357

Porter JM, Pidgeon C, Cunningham AJ. The sitting position in neurosurgery: a critical appraisal. *Br J Anaesth* 1999; 82(1): 117–128

5 Temperature control in theatre

Normal core body temperature of 37°C is controlled by the anterior hypothalamus via a number of mechanisms that modify heat production and loss.

Cold causes:

1 Shivering.
2 Stress hormone release.
3 Increased activity to increase heat production.
4 Cutaneous vasoconstriction.
5 Horripilation.
6 Behavioural adaptations to decrease heat loss.
7 Hunger.

During anaesthesia volatile and narcotic agents lower the basal metabolic rate, reset hypothalamic temperature control to lower than normal and cause vasodilatation. Muscle relaxants prevent shivering. Heat loss in theatre may be divided into:

- Radiant losses from the body (40%) that will be exacerbated by low environmental temperatures.
- Convection (30%) as the air around the body is warmed by conduction, expands and rises, drawing in colder air next to the skin.
- Evaporation (30%) from exposed skin, open body cavities and respiratory tract due to the latent heat of vaporization.

Cold intravenous fluid, wet drapes and cold anaesthetic gases all contribute to the problem. The very young and the very old are at greatest risk. The effects of hypothermia can be serious and include a fivefold increase in oxygen requirement due to shivering, myocardial depression with a risk of VF below 28°C, decreased level of consciousness, decreased drug metabolism and hyperglycaemia. Prevention involves planning ahead to provide:

- Monitoring of patient temperature at suitable site(s).
- A suitable environmental temperature.
- Warmed and humidified gases.
- Warmed intravenous fluids.
- Insulation.
- Active warming devices, including overhead radiant heaters for neonates when possible.

Further reading

Berti M, Fanelli G, Casati A, Aldegheri G, Lugani D, Torri G. Hypothermia prevention and treatment. *Anaesthesia* 1998; 53(Suppl): 246–247

Bock M, Muller J, Bach A, Bohrer H, Martin E, Motsch J. Effects of preinduction and intraoperative warming during major laparotomy. *Br J Anaesth* 1998; 80(2): 159–163

Desborough JP. Body temperature control and anaesthesia. *Br J Hosp Med* 1997; 57(9): 440–442

6 | Volume of distribution

The volume of distribution of a drug (Vd) is the apparent dilution space into which the drug distributes. This may correspond to a true physiological volume, but can be thought of as a proportionality constant which relates the quantity of drug in the body at any time to the plasma concentration at that time. The Vd therefore gives an idea of the extent of distribution of a drug:

$$Vd = \frac{Q}{C}$$

Q = amount of drug
C = concentration in plasma

A drug that is tightly bound to plasma proteins has a Vd of about 0.06 l kg^{-1}, which corresponds to the plasma volume per kg body weight. Experimentally, dyes such as Evans blue can be used to estimate plasma volume. Drugs that pass through the capillary endothelium, but not through cell membranes and which are not protein bound or lipid soluble, have a Vd of approximately 0.2 l kg^{-1}, corresponding to the extracellular fluid volume (ECF). Insulin, mannitol and thiocyanate can estimate the ECF. If the drug passes through cell membranes, but is not bound to any tissue constituent or sequestered into any compartment, it will be evenly distributed throughout body water and will have a Vd of approximately 0.6 l kg^{-1}. However, if a drug is selectively bound to constituents of tissues or is taken up selectively bound to constituents of tissues or is taken up selectively by tissue cells the Vd becomes much greater than any physiological volume. In summary, high values of Vd imply that the drug is accumulating in at least one tissue of the body and low values imply that the drug is remaining in the plasma.

Drugs confined to the plasma compartment

Drugs may be confined to the plasma compartment for two main reasons. Firstly, the drug molecules may be too large to cross the capillary wall easily, e.g. heparin. Secondly, the drug may be strongly bound to plasma proteins, e.g. phenylbutazone and warfarin.

Drugs distributed throughout total body water (TBW)

These drugs are highly lipid soluble and therefore cross cell membranes easily, including the blood–brain barrier and placental barrier. Examples include pentobarbitone, phenytoin, ethanol and diazepam. Drugs with very high values of Vd, greater than the estimated TBW (morphine, digoxin and haloperidol, for example) may be bound to sites anywhere outside the plasma compartment, or sequestered in fat.

Further reading

McLeod HL. Pharmacokinetics for the prescriber. *Medicine* 1999; 27: 10–14

Rowland M, Tozer TN. *Clinical Pharmacokinetics: Concepts and Applications*, 3rd edtion. Lea & Febiger, Philadelphia, 1995

7   Amiodarone

Amiodarone is a Class III anti-dysrrhythmic drug whose major indications include the treatment of a wide range of tachycardias, e.g. paroxysmal supraventricular tachycardias, nodal and ventricular tachycardias, atrial fibrillation and flutter and ventricular fibrillation which are resistant to other drugs. These include those associated with the Wolff–Parkinson–White syndrome. The mechanism of action is to increase the duration of the action potential in atrial and ventricular myocardium, prolonging the Q–T interval. The exact mechanism is not fully understood, but it is known to inhibit fast sodium channels and to affect repolarization by its effect on potassium channels. When given intravenously, amiodarone may also exhibit non-competitive α-blocking and mild negative inotropic effects. Coronary artery vasodilation may occur when given orally. Amiodarone has a very long half-life (may be weeks), which is particularly important where drug interactions are concerned. The administration of amiodarone intravenously is via a central line with a loading dose of 300 mg in 100 ml 5% dextrose given over 1–4 hours in an adult. A further 900 mg should be given over the next 18–24 hours to make a total of 1.2 g in 24 hours. It can then be given orally.

Amiodarone may become arrhythmogenic when given concurrently with drugs which also prolong the Q–T interval. The plasma levels of warfarin and digoxin are increased and their dose should be reduced by approximately half. Amiodarone has an additive effect with β-blockers and calcium channel blockers, resulting in an increased degree of nodal block. Side effects include nausea, photosensitivity, blue-grey skin discoloration, abnormalities of thyroid dysfunction, corneal microdeposits, peripheral neuropathy and pneumonitis.

Further reading

Hughes M, Binning A. Intravenous amiodarone in intensive care: time for a reappraisal? *Intensive Care Med* 2000; 26(12): 1730–1739

Larsen JA, Kadish AH, Schwartz JB. Proper use of antiarrhythmic therapy for reduction of mortality after myocardial infarction. *Drugs Aging* 2000; 16(5): 341–350

Nolan PE, Nappi J, Pollak PT. Clinical efficacy of amiodarone. *Pharmacotherapy* 1998; 18(6 Pt 2): 127S–137S

8 | Extracorporeal membrane oxygenation in neonates

Extracorporeal membrane oxygenation (ECMO) is a modified form of cardiopulmonary bypass that was first developed by Bartlett in 1976 to provide prolonged respiratory and/or cardiac support.

Using veno-arterial ECMO (see second figure), blood drains by gravity from the right atrium via a cannula placed in the right internal jugular vein and is returned using a roller pump, once oxygenated and warmed, to the aortic arch via a cannula placed in the common carotid artery. The use of ECMO requires systemic anticoagulation with heparin and haemorrhage (especially intracranial) constitutes the major complication of this therapy.

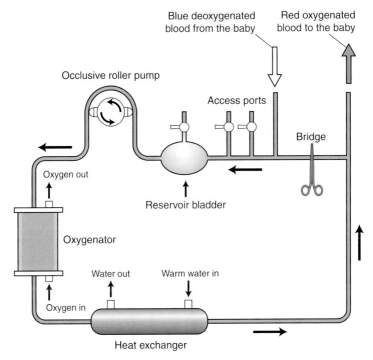

(After Dodds, with permission from Churchill Livingstone.)

The UK Collaborative Randomised Trial of Neonatal ECMO was a large controlled study of mature neonates with severe respiratory failure, comparing optimal conventional therapy with treatment in an ECMO centre. ECMO decreased mortality from 59% (54/93 children) to 32% (30/93 children). Follow-up at 1 year demonstrated no difference in neurological or respiratory disability between the two groups. An oxygenation index (OI) > 40 may be an indicator for ECMO if the following criteria are met:

127

- Gestation > 34 weeks.
- Weight > 2 kg.
- Reversible lung disease.
- No major intracranial haemorrhage.
- No lethal congenital anomalies.

Define oxygenation index:

$$OI = \frac{AWP \times FiO_2 \times 100}{PaO_2 \ (mmHg)}$$

where AWP = mean airway pressure.

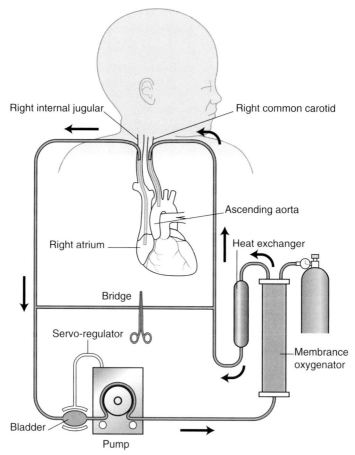

(After Flemming and Clutton-Brock, with permission from Churchill Livingstone.)

Further reading

Beardsmore C, Dundas I, Poole K, Enock K, Stocks J. Respiratory function in survivors of the United Kingdom Extracorporeal Membrane Oxygenation Trial. *Am J Respir Crit Care Med* 2000; 161(4 Pt 1): 1129–1135

Dodds C. Extracorporeal Membrane Oxygenation in neonates. *Curr Anaesth Crit Care* 1997; 8: 299

Fleming IMG, Clutton-Brock TH. Extracorporeal membrane oxygenation. *Curr Anaesth Crit Care* 1996; 7: 167–174

Kossel H, Bauer K, Kewitz G, Karaca S, Versmold H. Do we need new indications for ECMO in neonates pretreated with high-frequency ventilation and/or inhaled nitric oxide? *Intensive Care Med* 2000; 26(10): 1489–1495

Roy BJ, Rycus P, Conrad SA, Clark RH. The changing demographics of neonatal extracorporeal membrane oxygenation patients reported to the Extracorporeal Life Support Organization (ELSO) Registry. *Pediatrics* 2000; 106(6): 1334–1338

UK Collaborative Trial Group. UK Collaborative Randomised Trial of Neonatal ECMO. *Lancet* 1996; 348: 75–82

9 Lithium therapy and anaesthesia

Lithium carbonate is used in the management of manic depressive disorders. Its mode of action is unknown. Lithium is absorbed well from the gastrointestinal tract. It is water soluble and relies almost exclusively on renal excretion, so that lithium clearance correlates with creatinine clearance. In the body it is handled like sodium and potassium ions and, therefore, can have profound effects on electrolyte balance and metabolic processes. The therapeutic range is 0.8–1.2 mmol l^{-1}. Toxicity can occur above 1.5–2.0 mmol l^{-1}. The therapeutic window is small and levels should be monitored closely.

Problems

Side effects and signs of early toxicity include:

- Gastrointestinal symptoms such as nausea, vomiting and diarrhoea.
- Fine tremor.
- Polyuria and polydipsia.
- Weight gain.

These progress to muscle weakness, slurred speech, sleepiness and confusion. Severe toxicity results in convulsions and life-threatening coma. Reduced fluid intake (e.g. from preoperative starvation, vomiting and obtunded states), combined with the lithium-induced inability to compensate by concentrating urine output, can cause dehydration and precipitate toxicity. Renal function can be disturbed either by preoperative events or by surgery itself, and this too may cause lithium toxicity by accumulation. Lithium is potentiated by NSAIDs and thiazide diuretics. Conversely, lithium can potentiate the action of neuromuscular agents by inhibiting presynaptic synthesis of acetylcholine.

Management

In the elective situation lithium should be stopped 48–72 hours prior to surgery. Intravenous therapy should be considered. Dehydration must be avoided with appropriate fluid management. Restart lithium as soon as feasible (to prevent acute mania) provided that renal function and fluid and electrolyte balance are normal. In the emergency situation, signs of toxicity should be sought on a clinical basis. The use of neuromuscular agent should be carefully monitored, but, nevertheless, it may be necessary to provide a period of respiratory support postoperatively until power is regained. Minor toxicity should be treated with rehydration and mannitol to increase excretion. Loop and thiazide diuretics are contraindicated. Haemodialysis may be required in severe coma inducing toxicity. As it is largely distributed through the extracellular fluid, haemodialysis is effective in clearing lithium.

Further reading

Gitlin M. Lithium and the kidney: an updated review. *Drug Saf* 1999; 20(3): 231–243

Vipond AJ, Bakewell S, Telford R, Nicholls AJ. Lithium toxicity. *Anaesthesia* 1996; 51(12): 1156–1158

 The pathophysiology of drowning and the resuscitation of a victim of near-drowning

Near-drowning can be defined as initial survival following asphyxia during liquid immersion.

Pathophysiology

- Initial voluntary apnoea: the diving reflex in infants consists of apnoea, bradycardia and peripheral vasoconstriction following cold water immersion of the face.
- Breakpoint: involuntary inspiration and gasping causing water to enter the airways. Swallowing, vomiting and aspiration of vomit is common; Laryngeal spasm may occur and persist, causing asphyxia and death – dry drowning.
- Secondary apnoea.
- Further voluntary gasping and loss of consciousness.
- Cardiorespiratory arrest.

Water entering the lungs causes an increase in airway resistance and a decrease in lung compliance. Reflex pulmonary vasoconstriction occurs and surfactant is both diluted and denatured. Inflammatory reactions cause disruption of the alveolar capillary membrane and plasma-rich exudate leaks into the alveoli. This leads to widespread atelectasis and pulmonary oedema resulting in severe V/Q mismatch and hypoxaemia. Fresh water is quickly absorbed into the circulation from the alveoli. This may rarely lead to electrolyte disturbance or haemolysis. Sea water is hypertonic and draws large amounts of plasma into the alveoli.

Management

Basic resuscitation will follow the usual guidelines. The victims of near-drowning often vomit. Particular attention should be paid to possible spinal injuries; cervical spine injuries are the commonest. A detailed history of the mechanism of the injury should be obtained where possible. Useful information includes:

- Length of immersion.
- Immersion medium, e.g. salt or fresh water.
- Temperature of the water and the ambient temperature.
- Contamination of the water.
- Initial condition of the victim and response to resuscitation.
- The time of the first respiratory effort may indicate prognosis.

Full, advanced cardiorespiratory support should be instituted. Particular points are:

1 Cardiovascular support:
   (a) Check U & Es and osmolality and give isotonic fluids.
   (b) Investigate for haemolysis: free urinary or plasma haemoglobin.
   (c) Administer blood products as required.
   (d) Invasive monitoring if indicated.
   (e) Inotropes may be required.
   (f) Metabolic acidosis unresponsive to resuscitation may require bicarbonate.
2 Respiratory support:
   (a) Give oxygen.
   (b) Chest and spinal X-ray.
   (c) Intubate and ventilate if airway compromised or casualty hypoxic.
   (d) Nasogastric tube required since there will be large volumes of swallowed water.
   (e) PEEP or CPAP may be helpful with pulmonary oedema.
3 Temperature control:
   (a) Hypothermia should be treated with slow rewarming over a number of hours using warming blankets, warmed fluids and warmed respiratory gases.
   (b) Very occasionally, invasive methods such as peritoneal lavage or cardiopulmonary bypass may be required.
4 Cerebral protection:
   (a) Ensure free venous drainage, mild hypocapnia and good blood pressure control.
   (b) Maintain normoglycaemia.
   (c) Decrease oxygen requirements by controlling fits and maintaining normothermia.
   (d) Consider intracranial pressure monitoring.
5 Microbiology: culture stomach and tracheal aspirates if the water was polluted.

Further reading

Ender PT, Dolan MJ. Pneumonia associated with near-drowning. *Clin Infect Dis* 1997; 25(4): 896–907

Giesbrecht GG. Cold stress, near drowning and accidental hypothermia: a review. *Aviat Space Environ Med* 2000; 71(7): 733–752

Zuckerman GB, Gregory PM, Santos-Damiani SM. Predictors of death and neurologic impairment in pediatric submersion injuries. The Pediatric Risk of Mortality Score. *Arch Pediatr Adolesc Med* 1998; 152(2): 134–140

11   The transurethral resection of prostate (TURP) syndrome

Pathophysiology

Transurethral resection of the prostate requires a non-conductive, non-electrolytic fluid with good optical properties to provide continuous irrigation. An isotonic 1.5% glycine solution is normally used. During resection prostatic venous sinuses are opened and since the hydrostatic pressure of irrigating fluid is higher than venous pressure, fluid enters the circulation at a rate of 20–60 ml min^{-1}. This results in volume overload, dilutional hyponatraemia and a relatively smaller drop in osmolality.

The risk factors are:

- Cardiovascular state.
- Length of resection and irrigation.
- Height of irrigation fluid.
- Vascularity of prostate.
- Head-down tilt.

Presentation

Initial manifestations are hypervolaemia with an increase in systolic blood pressure and pulse pressure and a bradycardia. Hypotension and cardiovascular collapse follow. This sequence may be masked by concurrent blood loss. Pulmonary oedema may occur with respiratory distress and cyanosis. Headache, confusion, convulsions and coma occur progressively as the sodium concentration falls and cerebral oedema develops. Glycine itself is an inhibitory neurotransmitter and may contribute to these symptoms along with one of its metabolites, ammonia.

Investigation

- Plasma sodium and osmolality.
- Haemoglobin and clotting profile if indicated.
- Glycine levels are occasionally indicated.

Management

- Reduce risk factors by limiting resection to 1 hour and irrigate with saline postoperatively. Limit irrigating pressure to 60 cm H_2O.
- Employing regional rather than general anaesthesia may allow the syndrome to be recognized earlier.

- Conservative treatment may be appropriate in asymptomatic patients and requires fluid restriction only. However, TURP syndrome is a cause of mortality and each case must be judged individually.
- Symptoms or very deranged results can be treated with normal saline and loop diuretics. Only rarely is it necessary to employ hypertonic saline and then great care must be taken to avoid over-rapid correction of hyponatraemia and risk central pontine myelinolysis. A rise of 2 mmol l^{-1} each hour is regarded as safe and the hypertonic saline should be stopped when serum sodium reaches 125 mmol l^{-1}.
- A very severely affected patient may need full intensive measures including IPPV, inotropes and ICP monitoring.

Further reading

Gehring H, Nahm W, Baerwald J et al. Irrigation fluid absorption during transurethral resection of the prostate: spinal vs. general anaesthesia. *Acta Anaesthesiol Scand* 1999; 43(4): 458–463

Gravenstein D. Transurethral resection of the prostate (TURP) syndrome: a review of the pathophysiology and management. *Anesth Analg* 1997; 84(2): 438–446

Heidler H. Frequency and causes of fluid absorption: a comparison of three techniques for resection of the prostate under continuous pressure monitoring. *BJU Int* 1999; 83(6): 619–622

12 The cleaning and sterilization of anaesthetic equipment

Although disposable equipment is increasingly being employed in anaesthetic practice, a number of items, such as laryngeal masks, are reusable and require appropriate cleaning to reduce the risk of cross-infection. The new menace of Creutzfeldt-Jacob disease will result in alterations in these recommendations but full details are as yet unavailable. At the present time there are three levels of cleaning equipment.

Decontamination

This involves washing and scrubbing to physically remove particles of matter and may be sufficient in itself and otherwise is an essential prerequisite to further processes.

Disinfection

This achieves the destruction of most infective organisms, but not spores. It is adequate for most purposes and suitable for perishable materials that cannot withstand the higher temperatures used during sterilization. Pasteurization involves heating the article in a water bath at 70°C for 20 minutes or 80°C for 10 minutes. Boiling for 5 minutes is effective. Both these methods require strict adherence to the temperatures and time required without adding extra articles in the middle of a cycle. There are a number of chemical disinfectants that may be employed in liquid form or, less commonly, as mists and fogs. Examples include chorhexidene used in varying concentrations; 2% glutaraldehyde, which is often used for endoscopic instruments and is rather toxic; and sodium hypochlorite. The latter is useful because it has a high antiviral activity but it corrodes metal.

Sterilization

Autoclaving is the most efficient means of sterilizing. The equipment is exposed to steam under increased pressure in a special sealed unit so that temperatures of over 130°C are reached. The process is automatically controlled, ensuring appropriate temperature, pressure and time and ending the cycle with a vacuum stage to remove moisture.

Dry heating at 150–160°C for 20–30 minutes is suitable for glass syringes and some metal instruments. Sterilization with ethylene oxide is technically difficult and expensive, but effective. This process uses a special chamber to control temperature and humidity and employs a 5–10% mixture. An elution period of 7–10 days is required following sterilization.

Gamma irradiation is generally used in the sterilization of large quantities of disposable goods and is not used in the hospital setting.

Further reading

Frosh A. Prions and the ENT surgeon. *J Laryngol Otol* 1999; 113(12): 1064–1067

Rutala WA, Weber DJ. Creutzfeldt–Jakob disease: recommendations for disinfection and sterilization. *Clin Infect Dis* 2001; 32(9): 1348–1356

Trasancos CC, Kainer MA, Desmond PV, Kelly H. Investigation of potential iatrogenic transmission of hepatitis C in Victoria, Australia. *Aust NZ J Public Health* 2001; 25(3): 241–244

Zobeley E, Flechsig E, Cozzio A, Enari M, Weissmann C. Infectivity of scrapie prions bound to a stainless steel surface. *Mol Med* 1999; 5(4): 240–243

Paper Two Write short notes on the following topics. Do not miss out any questions and remember that there are only 3 hours in total to complete this paper.

1 The anatomy and relationships of the diaphragm
2 Monoamine oxidase inhibitors and anaesthesia
3 Alveolar hypoventilation: its causes and relevance to pulse oximetry
4 The APACHE scoring system
5 The discharge criteria for day-stay patients
6 The adverse effects of nitrous oxide (N_2O)
7 Acute major anaphylaxis
8 The diagnosis of brain death
9 The clinical uses of capnography
10 The management of postdural puncture headache
11 The concentration and second gas effects
12 What are possible contraindications to the use of an arterial tourniquet?

Paper Two

The anatomy and relationships of the diaphragm

The diaphragm is a fibromuscular sheet which separates the thorax from the abdomen. The peripheral part is muscular: the central part is aponeurotic and is called the central tendon. During inspiration the diaphragm flattens and descends vertically. During expiration it relaxes and returns to its previous position by lung recoil and the action of the abdominal muscles. The central tendon is fused with the undersurface of the pericardium.

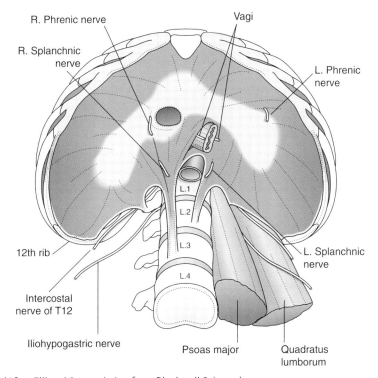

(After Ellis, with permission from Blackwell Science.)

Peripheral attachments are:

1 A *vertebral part* arising from the crura and from the arcuate ligaments. The arcuate ligaments are a series of fibrous arches, the medial overlying and attaching to quadratus lumborum. Attached to the vertebrae (upper 3 lumbar on right, upper 2 lumbar on left) are the right and left crura, which lie between the medial arches. The fibrous medial borders of the two crura form the medium arcuate ligament over the front of the aorta.

2   A *costal part* attached to the inner aspect of the lower six ribs and costal cartilages.

3   A *sternal part* consisting of two small slips from the deep surface of the xiphisternum.

There are three main openings:

1   For the *aorta* (at T12), which also transmits the thoracic duct and azygos vein.

2   For the *oesophagus* (at T10), which penetrates the muscular fibres above the right crus and also various branches of the left gastric artery and the two vagi.

3   For the *inferior vena cava* (at T8), in the central tendon, which also transmits the right phrenic nerve.

The diaphragm is also pierced by the left phrenic nerve (in the central tendon) and the splanchnic nerves, which pass through the right and left crura. The sympathetic chain passes behind the diaphragm deep to the medial arcuate ligament. The nerve supply is from C3–5 via the phrenic nerves with some sensory supply to the periphery via the lower intercostal nerves.

Further reading

Ellis H. *Clinical Anatomy*. Blackwell Science, Oxford, 1996.

2   Monoamine oxidase inhibitors and anaesthesia

Monoamine oxidase inhibitors (MAOIs) still have a definite and probably increasing role in the management of depression. Monoamine oxidase (MAO) is one of the two main enzymes involved in the inactivation of non-methylated biogenic amines and is found inside adrenergic neurones. Here it controls the level of free noradrenaline available for release into the synaptic cleft. Inhibition of the action of MAO by an MAOI leads to a greater mobile pool of noradrenaline in the presynaptic nerve ending.

Mechanism of action

MAOIs act by forming a stable, irreversible complex with MAO, mainly in cerebral neurones and also in the sympathetic nervous system, gut and liver. Since the majority of MAOIs cause irreversible enzyme inhibition, their effects are prolonged and last for several weeks. A new class of antibiotics, oxazolidinones (Linezolid) have minor MAOI effects.

Side effects

MAOIs traditionally carry a bad reputation in anaesthesia. This is based principally on early reports of interaction with pethidine, which has brought other opioids under suspicion. Interaction with opioids may be excitatory or depressive. The *excitatory* form is characterized by agitation, difficult behaviour, headache, hyperreflexia, rigidity, hyper- or hypotension and coma. It is thought to be due to excessive central serotonin activity and has only been reported with pethidine, which reduces serotonin uptake from nerve endings. This response to pethidine is frequently severe and can be fatal. The *depressive* form produces respiratory depression, hypotension and unconsciousness. It is thought to be the result of hepatic enzyme inhibition by the MAOI increasing the serum level of narcotic.

Sympathomimetic drugs may produce exaggerated hypertensive responses, particularly those such as ephedrine, amphetamine and metaraminol, which in part act indirectly by releasing noradrenaline from nerve terminals.

Management

Morphine (in a reduced dosage) has been established as a safe drug in these patients and is the narcotic of choice for both elective and emergency surgery. The patient does, however, need careful monitoring in case of a depressive reaction. Naloxone should be readily available and noradrenaline (in very carefully titrated doses) can be used as a vasopressor to reverse hypotension. If sympathomimetics are necessary, directly acting drugs such as adrenaline, noradrenaline and isoprenaline are the more reliable. It is recommended that adrenaline-containing solutions of local anaesthetic should be avoided. Nitrous oxide, halothane, enflurane and isoflurane are all safe in the presence of MAOIs. Phenelzine decreases plasma cholinesterase and may prolong the action of suxamethonium. Ketamine theoretically should be avoided in patients on MAOIs although there are no adverse reports in the literature. The concurrent use of benzodiazepines is usually considered safe. Because of the long-term action of MAOIs and the risk of depression if they are stopped very early before elective surgery, it has been recommended (because there are safe anaesthetic regimens which can be given) that the old custom of stopping the drugs well before elective surgery is discontinued. In patients on MAOIs treatment should continue as normal until the day of surgery.

Further reading

Smith MS, Muir H, Hall R. Perioperative management of drug therapy, clinical considerations. *Drugs* 1996; 51(2): 238–259

Stack CG, Rogers P, Linter SPK. Monoamine oxidase inhibitors and anaesthesia. *Br J Anaesth* 1998; 60: 222–227

---

3   Alveolar hypoventilation: its causes and relevance to pulse oximetry

Alveolar hypoventilation can result from:

1   Chronic obstructive airways disease.
2   Impaired mechanical ventilation (acute airways obstruction, stiff lungs, flail chest, pneumothorax, underventilation, disconnection).

3 Muscular weakness (myopathy, neuropathy, relaxant drugs).

4 Central depression from drugs (opioids, sedatives, anaesthetic agents).

In a conscious person, if the failure of alveolar ventilation is secondary to chronic abnormal neuromuscular function or the residual effects of sedative drugs, the patient may show little distress: if it is secondary to a mechanical problem he will make vigorous efforts to increase his tidal and minute volumes.

When alveolar hypoventilation occurs there is insufficient gas movement to both oxygenate the blood and to wash out the carbon dioxide, so the PaO_2 is reduced and the $PaCO_2$ is elevated. In the presence of alveolar hypoventilation the PaO_2 (but not the $PaCO_2$) can be greatly improved by increasing the inspired oxygen concentration.

Pulse oximetry measures the saturation of oxygen in the arterial blood. Its relation to the oxygen content is described by the sigmoid oxyhaemoglobin dissociation curve. The saturation will therefore variably indicate the degree of oxygen tension as determined by the part of the curve it is on. At acceptable levels of oxygen saturation, there has to be a large change in the PaO_2 to produce a detectable change on a pulse oximeter. At lower saturations a small change in PaO_2 will be seen as a major change in saturation value.

While breathing spontaneously under the influence of anaesthetics or in the postoperative recovery period, patients have an impaired response to a rising $PaCO_2$ and alveolar hypoventilation results. In the presence of alveolar hypoventilation, if the patient is breathing room air the saturation will fall relatively early and the pulse oximeter will indicate inadequate function in terms of oxygenation. Usually in recovery the patient is receiving supplemental oxygen with an inspired oxygen concentration well above 20%. Under these conditions, the alveolar PaO_2 will remain elevated, as will the saturation and the alveolar $PaCO_2$ levels will have to rise much further before peripheral hypoxaemia occurs. The saturation gives no indication of hypoventilation. There have been several cases reported of severe hypercarbia produced by this mechanism. It is important to remember that the pulse oximeter measures peripheral oxygen saturation: *it is not a measure of adequacy of ventilation and gives no indication of the level of the $PaCO_2$.*

Further reading

Hutton P, Clutton-Brock TH. The benefits and pitfalls of pulse oximetry. *BMJ* 1993; 307: 457–458

Nunn JF. *Applied Respiratory Physiology*, 4th edition. Butterworth Heinemann, Oxford, 1993: 258

4   The APACHE scoring system

APACHE is an acronym for acute physiology and chronic health evaluation, and is one of a number of scoring systems used to try to predict outcome from intensive care. It was also intended to allow stratification of patients into groups to compare different therapies. The original system (APACHE I, 1981) had 34 variables which were assigned weighted values by an expert panel of physicians depending upon their deviation above or below the normal range. The large number of variables made the score cumbersome to use and several of the variables were found not to increase the predictive power of the index. It was modified, simplified and reintroduced in 1985 as APACHE II, which uses 12 variables that have been shown to have a bearing on outcome. With these modifications, the APACHE II system generated a single score (the level of which increased with severity of illness) from three sources:

1 The acute physiology score (12 variables in total): 10 physiological variables (0–4 points), creatinine (0–8 points), Glasgow coma scale (0–12 points).

2 Age points (0–6).

3 Chronic health points (0–5).

This generates a maximum of 71 points.

The score provides a working indication of severity of illness and is therefore a common language. Attempts have been made to develop it further. By combining this score with a stratified index of the admission diagnosis an estimate of the risk of death was derived. Validation has been attempted on many thousands of patients.

In summary, although on grouped data prediction is good, because of the widely differing prognoses of different diseases it is not possible to estimate a patient's risk of hospital mortality using APACHE II admission scores alone. Two patients with the same admission scores, but from different causes (e.g. severe diabetic coma, septic shock), are likely to have very different outcomes. In using age, chronic disease, acute physiology, diagnosis and surgical status to predict the risk of death, the APACHE II system maximizes the use of patient data to form prognoses: the other major determinant of outcome, the response to treatment (which is disease specific), has been addressed by other systems and is included in the son of APACHE II, APACHE III.

Further reading

Knaus WA, Draper EA, Wagner DP, Zimmerman JE. APACHE II: a severity of disease classification. *Crit Care Med* 1985; 13: 818–829

Riddington DW, Clutton-Brook TH. Monitoring the severity of illness. In: Hutton P, Prys Robers C, eds. *Monitoring in Anaesthesia and Intensive Care*. Saunders, London 1994; 415–424

5 The discharge criteria for day-stay patients

Day care is a rapidly evolving area of practice and hence the guidelines are changing as the scope of day care widens but the fundamental principles remain the same. Postoperative assessment must be performed before discharge by an experienced anaesthetist. Although the details differ from publication to publication, the following represents a typical list of requirements:

1 Full orientation and responsiveness.
2 Ability to walk and dress with full coordination.
3 Ability to drink and speak properly.
4 No uncontrolled surgical factors (e.g. bleeding, swelling).
5 Stable vital signs.
6 Adequately controlled pain and instructions concerning further analgesia.
7 Appropriate transport home accompanied by a responsible person.
8 Appropriate, non-isolated home conditions.
9 Written and verbal instructions not to take depressant drugs or alcohol or to undertake potentially self-damaging activities (e.g. driving, operating machinery), for 24 hours.
10 A contact number in case of distress.
11 Minimal nausea and vomiting.

Further reading

Beauregard L, Pomp A, Choiniere M. Severity and impact of pain after day-surgery. *Can J Anaesth* 1998; 45(4): 304–311

Eger EI, White PF, Bogetz MS. Clinical and economic factors important to anaesthetic choice for day-case surgery. *Pharmacoeconomics* 2000; 17(3): 245–262

Korttila K. Recovery from outpatient anaesthesia: factors affecting outcome. *Anaesthesia* 1995; 50(Suppl): 22–28

Tzabar Y, Asbury AJ, Millar K. Cognitive failures after general anaesthesia for day-case surgery. *Br J Anaesth* 1996; 76(2): 194–197

Wedderburn AW, Dodds SR, Morris GE. A survey of post-operative care after day case surgery. *Ann R Coll Surg Engl* 1996; 78(2 Suppl): 70–71

---

6   **The adverse effects of nitrous oxide (N_2O)**

In summary, these are problems with:

- Diffusion.
- Nausea and vomiting.
- Combustion.
- Increases in cerebral blood flow.
- Risk of hypoxic mixtures.
- Influence on vitamin B_{12}.

Diffusion effects: as N_2O is more soluble than nitrogen, when inhaled nitrogen is replaced with N_2O, the volume or pressure of gas-filled cavities will increase. This may be of particular relevance in pneumothorax or intracranial air (following either trauma or surgery) where a rapid rise in volume may lead to a tension pneumothorax or increased intracranial pressure. Following the discontinuation of N_2O at the end of anaesthesia, there is rapid excretion of N_2O into the lungs, with the risk of diffusion hypoxia. This can be minimized by the use of face mask oxygen for 15 minutes in recovery. There is the ever present risk of administering a hypoxic gas mixture to a patient. Therefore inspired oxygen monitoring is essential when N_2O is being used. In the UK it should now be impossible to administer N_2O without a minimum oxygen mixture.

Teratogenicity: short-term exposure in the first trimester of pregnancy is safe, as is low-level exposure in properly scavenged anaesthetic rooms. However, a reduction in fertility and an increase in miscarriages have been reported in dental assistants, where N_2O was not scavenged.

Postoperative nausea and vomiting may be increased with the use of N_2O. The effect is probably due to several factors including middle ear pressure changes, gastric distension, sympathomimetic effects and opioid receptor stimulation.

As N_2O supports combustion, there is a risk of airway fire during laser surgery. The avoidance of N_2O with an air/oxygen mixture may be safer. N_2O causes a small reduction in cardiac index used in conjunction with volatile agents.

N_2O is said to increase cerebral blood flow. The increase is greater with isoflurane/N_2O mixtures than with isoflurane alone. Some anaesthetists would therefore avoid N_2O in the presence of raised intracranial pressure or intracranial air.

Vitamin B_{12} is a cofactor for the enzyme methionine synthetase, which is essential for the conversion of homocysteine to methionine and the production of thymidine for DNA synthesis. Inhibition of the former leads to methionine deficiency, which can cause subacute combined degeneration of the spinal cord and peripheral neuropathy. It is the inhibition of DNA synthesis that causes megaloblastic bone marrow depression. The inhibition of DNA synthesis has led to concerns about teratogenicity. N_2O irreversibly inactivates vitamin B_{12}, leading to an inhibition of methionine synthetase and DNA synthesis.

Further reading

Brownlie GS, Walters FJM. Should we still be using nitrous oxide? *Curr Anaesth Crit Care* 1994; 5: 109–114

Kolbitsch C, Lorenz I, Keller C, Schmidauer C, Hormann C, Benzer A. The influence of increasing concentrations of nitrous oxide on cerebral blood flow velocity in hypocapnic patients with brain tumours. *Eur J Anaesthesiol* 1999; 16(8): 543–546

McKinney MS, Fee JP. Cardiovascular effects of 50% nitrous oxide in older adult patients anaesthetized with isoflurane or halothane. *Br J Anaesth* 1998; 80(2): 169–173

7 Acute major anaphylaxis

Acute major anaphylaxis is an uncommon (1:4000) but well recognized and potentially fatal, complication of anaesthesia. The management of a severe episode can be divided into three phases:

Immediate management

Stop giving the suspect drug, summon help, discontinue surgery and anaesthesia if feasible, intubate the patient and start IPPV with 100% oxygen, give adrenaline (1 ml of 1:10 000 aliquots as required), give colloid (10 ml kg^{-1} and repeat as necessary) and consider external cardiac massage. Several litres of colloid (ideally albumin solution) may be required. Adrenaline should be used early, repeatedly and by infusion if necessary, to maintain an adequate arterial blood pressure.

Secondary management

Give steroids for bronchospasm or cardiovascular collapse. For persistent bronchospasm consider β_2-adrenoceptor agonists or aminophylline. Ketamine or volatile anaesthetic agents may occasionally help in severe bronchospasm. For intractable severe bronchospasm, consider external chest compression and cardiopulmonary bypass. Give chlorpheniramine as well as type 2 histamine receptor blockers. Consider sodium bicarbonate if a severe metabolic acidosis persists. Take blood for clotting screen, electrolytes, arterial blood gases and mast cell tryptase. Collect urine for methylhistamine measurement.

Tertiary management

After 4–6 weeks the patient should be reviewed. Skin testing should be considered in all patients following a suspected major anaphylactic reaction. A letter should be given to the patient detailing the nature of the reaction, the drugs involved and the results of investigations. If further anaesthetics are administered, the results of these should be added to the letter. Patients should be encouraged to wear a warning device such as a Medic Alert bracelet. Every department should display an algorithm for the management of major acute anaphylaxis wherever anaesthesia is undertaken.

Further reading

Anaphylactic Reactions Associated with Anaesthesia. Association of Anaesthetists, London 1995

Fisher MMcD, Baldo BA. Anaphylactoid reactions during anaesthesia. In: Atkinson RS, Adams AP (eds). *Recent Advances in Anaesthesia and Analgesia*, Vol. 18. Churchill Livingstone, London, 1994: 159–177

8 The diagnosis of brain death

This is now synonymous with death of the brainstem. The irreversible cessation of brainstem function implies death of the brain as a whole. It does not necessarily imply the immediate death of every cell in the brain. The diagnosis of brainstem death depends upon:

1 Essential preconditions.
2 Necessary exclusions.
3 Tests of brainstem function.

Essential preconditions

Two preconditions are necessary: firstly that the patient is in apnoeic coma, i.e. unresponsive and on a ventilator; and secondarily that the cause of the coma is irremediable brain damage, i.e. no treatment may change the outcome of the condition.

Necessary exclusions

Drug intoxication, hypothermia and metabolic and endocrine disturbances can all cause profound yet reversible changes in brainstem function and need to be excluded. Physiological parameters such as blood pressure, temperature and electrolytes should all be within acceptable limits.

Tests of brainstem function

The loss of brainstem function is diagnosed on the basis of:

(a) Coma.
(b) No abnormal postures, facial movements or epileptiform jerking.
     If present, these features imply the passage of nervous impulses through functioning cells in the brain stem.
(c) No brainstem reflexes. There are five brainstem reflexes to be assessed. For the diagnosis of a non-functioning brain stem there must be:
     (i)   No pupillary response to light.
     (ii) No corneal reflex.
     (iii) No vestibulo-ocular reflexes.
     (iv) No motor responses within the cranial nerve distribution (grimacing) in response to adequate stimulation (deliberate somatic pain).
     (v)   No gag or other reflex response to bronchial stimulation (passage of suction catheter).
(d) No spontaneous respiration.

Apnoea is established by showing that no respiratory movements occur when the patient is disconnected from the ventilator at levels of arterial carbon

dioxide tension which would stimulate vigorous respiration in the normal patient
– over 6.65 kPa (50 mmHg).

Virtually all the codes published recommend that testing be carried out twice.
This ensures that there is no observer error and that there is no change in the
clinical signs.

Doll eye movement testing is not part of the UK code but is a useful test to do
early, because if the response is positive the brainstem is still alive and further
testing is unnecessary.

Further reading

Pallis C. *ABC of Brain Stem Death*. British Medical Journal, London, 1989

---

9 **The clinical uses of capnography**

Capnography measures the partial pressure of carbon dioxide in the gaseous
phase such as expired gas.

1 In patients with normal respiratory and cardiovascular systems it can be
   used as a non-invasive, breath-by-breath estimator of the $PaCO_2$. It thus
   allows ventilation to normocapnia without recourse to arterial blood gas
   measurement. The occurrence of a steeply sloping plateau denotes a spread
   of V/Q ratios and the greater the slope, the greater the alveolar dead space.
   Under these conditions, blood gases are required to confirm ventilation to
   normocapnia.

2 It can give qualitative evidence that rebreathing is occurring by the
   measurement of the minimum inspired concentration of CO_2.

3 It can be used to act as an apnoea alarm and hence as a disconnection
   alarm during IPPV.

4 It can, under certain circumstances, act as a disconnection monitor during
   spontaneous breathing. If the fresh gas supply fails and rebreathing
   occurs the $PiCO_2$ will rise steadily, indicating rebreathing. If the breathing
   circuit together with the sampling port becomes disconnected from the
   patient, apnoea will be shown. If, however, the sampling port remains
   connected to the endotrocheal tube, face or face mask, the only signs will
   be those related to the lightening of anaesthesia such as changing
   respiratory rate or pattern.

5 Although its use to measure respiratory rate is trivial during IPPV, during
   spontaneous breathing the respiratory rate can be a useful guide to the
   adequacy of anaesthesia and fresh gas flow.

6 A sudden fall in the $PetCO_2$ (i.e. occurring progressively breath by breath
   over a minute or so) indicates a sudden reduction of blood flow to ventilated
   lung tissue, which is usually expressed in the textbooks as a 'sudden increase
   in physiological dead space'. This is most likely to be caused by some form of
   air embolism or impending or actual cardiac arrest.

7   In the presence of alveolar ventilation, more gradual and less dramatic falls in the $PetCO_2$ may indicate hyperventilation, hypothermia, a reduction in the circulating fluid volume, hypotension or a reduction in the rate of production of CO_2.

8   An increase in the $PetCO_2$ during constant ventilation can be due to underventilation, rebreathing or an increase in CO_2 delivery to the lung (e.g. rapid blood transfusion). A significant and progressive rise in the $PetCO_2$ occurring when the ventilation should be adequate has also been recorded as one of the first signs of malignant hyperthermia.

9   The capnograph has been recommended as a device to confirm placement of endotrocheal tube in the trachea following a difficult intubation. The presence of CO_2 in the expired gas is not adequate to confirm placement since the stomach contains gas which may be in gaseous equilibrium with the tissues. It is essential that the shape of the capnograph is inspected. If it is abnormal, and/or if the maximum PCO_2 decreases rapidly with each breath, then oesophageal intubation must be assumed to be the most likely cause.

10   The onset of a notch in the alveolar plateau can indicate that the patient is trying to breathe spontaneously against the ventilator.

11   In circle systems the capnograph can indicate exhaustion of the soda lime. This will be seen initially as a rise in the minimum inspired concentration of CO_2 and later as a rise in the end-tidal value.

Abbreviations: CO_2 = carbon dioxide, $PaCO_2$ = arterial CO_2, $PiCO_2$ = inspired CO_2, $PetCO_2$ = end-tidal CO_2.

Further reading

Gravenstein JS, Paulus DA, Hayes TJ. *Capnography in Clinical Practice.* Butterworths, Boston, MA, 1989

Hardwick M, Hutton P. Capnography: fundamentals of current clinical practice. *Curr Anaesth Crit Care* 1990; 1: 176–180

10   The management of postdural puncture headache

Postdural puncture headache (PDPH) occurs as a result of intentional dural puncture for spinal anaesthesia, after lumbar puncture to obtain cerebrospinal fluid or to inject contrast media for myelogram and from unintentional puncture during epidural space location. The likelihood of headache occurring is greatest when large needles of Quincke design produce a dural hole in young ambulant patients. The obstetric population is especially vulnerable.

The first aspect of management is recognizing that the headache is as a result of dural puncture. Besides a temporal relationship to known or suspected dural puncture (the headache normally occurs within 24 hours although can present later) the important clinical feature is that of the headache being relieved by recumbency and exacerbated by standing. Where doubt exists, the headache can also be relieved dramatically by firm lower abdominal pressure (Gutsche sign).

A PDPH can be severe and debilitating. The management options are:

1 Prophylactic bed rest. This merely delays the onset of headache and hence is not recommended.
2 Increased hydration. This has little or no effect on subsequent headache.
3 Wait for spontaneous resolution. The headache will usually resolve within 2 or 3 days but may last up to 10 days. Unless the headache is mild this may not be acceptable.
4 Oral analgesics may help but do not usually cure the PDPH.
5 Abdominal binders can help but are not popular.
6 Caffeine therapy. This can be given orally (300 mg) or intravenously (500 mg) and is beneficial in reducing PDPH.
7 Oral theophylline (300 mg) in a sustained-release tablet has also been reported to ameliorate PDPH.
8 Epidural saline infusions: saline (1–1.5 litres) is infused over 24 hours into the epidural space. This has largely been superseded by epidural blood patch.
9 Epidural blood patch: autologous blood (15–20 ml) is injected into the epidural space near the dural puncture site under aseptic conditions. It has a high success rate, with the PDPH resolving within minutes normally. It may be repeated for severe refractory headaches.
10 Epidural Dextran 40: 30–40 ml is injected in a similar way to an epidural blood patch, with relief occurring within 2 hours. This may be suitable for patients where autologous blood is contraindicated or unacceptable.

11   The concentration and second gas effects

The concentration effect describes the process by which higher concentrations of inhaled anaesthetics reach a given proportion of their inspired concentration (Fi) in the alveoli (Fa) earlier than a lower concentration would; i.e. if a patient could breathe 60% or 6% of a given agent, his alveolar/inspiratory concentration ratio would reach 30%/40% before it reached 3%/6%. There are two reasons for this.

After a few breaths, a high inspired agent concentration will result in a rapid increase in the alveolar concentration. As non-agent-containing blood meets the agent-filled alveoli, there will be an uptake dependent upon the concentration gradient: this uptake will, however, still leave a relatively high concentration in the alveoli which will continue to drive the agent transfer. In addition, imagine that a patient breathing air is suddenly connected to a reservoir bag containing 75% N_2O and 25% O_2 at an atmospheric pressure of 101 kPa and within a few breaths the concentration of N_2O in the alveoli is 50% (approx 50.5 kPa). Initially the blood perfusing these alveoli would have no N_2O dissolved and, assuming the blood/gas partition coefficient to be 0.47, blood equilibrating with the alveoli would take up $(0.47 \times 50.5/101) = 0.235$ litres of N_2O per litre of blood. With a cardiac output of 5 l min^{-1}, every minute 1.175 litres of N_2O would be taken up. Consequently, each expired tidal volume would be less than each inspired total volume by 1.175 litres divided by the respiratory rate per minute. The difference between inspired and expired volumes would be greater the higher the concentration of N_2O in the inspired gas. Theoretically, the alveolar volume would gradually reduce and alveolar collapse would occur. This is of course not what happens because, being an open system, as the N_2O is taken up more fresh gas flows down the breathing system and bronchial tree to replace it. There is, because of gas uptake in the lung, increased effective alveolar ventilation.

The net effect of these processes, in which alveolar ventilation is increased by an amount dependent upon the net uptake of anaesthetic gas – the rate of which is also dependent upon the fractional concentration of the gas itself – is known as the concentration effect. In summary, a lower inspired N_2O level not only has lower proportionate value in the alveoli but it reaches that value and approaches final equilibrium more slowly. The knock-on effect of the net uptake of N_2O producing an effective increase in alveolar ventilation (which occurs in an ever-decreasing way until the patient's blood N_2O tension is in equilibrium with that in the alveoli) causes the partial pressure of oxygen in the alveoli to rise because more oxygen enters the alveoli, while the uptake of oxygen remains constant. The PaO_2 therefore rises because of the high uptake of N_2O and this is called the second gas effect. It occurs whenever one component of a gas mixture is replaced by a soluble gas and ventilation and circulation continue. If a third component in the form of a volatile agent is present, its alveolar concentration will also theoretically be increased.

12 **What are possible contraindications to the use of an arterial tourniquet?**

1   Severe peripheral vascular disease (may produce permanent ischaemia or damage to 'pipe-stem' arteries).

2   Sickle cell disease (may precipitate sickling).

3   Severe arthritis in the limb, or a recent fracture (may distort bones going to the adjacent joint or load a weak bone).

4   Badly injured limb (may confuse adequacy of blood supply).

5   Major coagulation disorders (may bruise badly under tourniquet or bleed on reperfusion).

6   Deep vein thrombosis in the limb.

7   Peripheral neuropathy or CNS defect affecting the limb (may compress inflamed nerves or cause confusion in diagnosis of post-tourniquet syndrome).

8   Poor skin condition of involved limb or very fragile skin, e.g. some premature babies, patients on steroids, the elderly and malnourished (may lead to blisters or skin damage).

9   Significant infection proximal to the tourniquet (may cause transfer of bacteria into general circulation).

Further reading

Kam PC, Kavanaugh R, Yoong FF. The arterial tourniquet: pathophysiological consequences and anaesthetic implications. *Anaestheisia* 2001; 56: 534–545

Write short notes on the following topics. Do not miss out any questions and remember that there are only 3 hours in total to complete this paper.

1 How does malignant hyperthermia present? Summarize how a case should be managed

2 Summarize the aetiology, presentation and physiological consequences of aortic stenosis

3 Anaesthesia for magnetic resonance imaging (MRI)

4 Critical temperature, critical pressure, isotherms and triple point

5 Causes of lactic acidosis

6 The functional residual capacity (FRC)

7 Endothelial derived relaxant factor (EDRF) – NO

8 Anaesthetic problems in acromegaly

9 Suxamethonium apnoea

10 Damage to the brachial plexus under general anaesthesia

11 The renin–angiotensin system

12 Pulmonary barotrauma

1 How does malignant hyperthermia present? Summarize how a case should be managed

The malignant hyperthermia (MH) syndrome is caused by a deficiency in the reuptake of calcium ions by the sarcoplasmic reticulum, which results in a failure of muscle relaxation following contraction. Consequently, muscle contraction is sustained, the rate of metabolism increases dramatically and the clinical MH syndrome develops. Although the condition usually presents intraoperatively, if the operation is short and the onset delayed, signs may not be apparent until the patient is in recovery or even back on the ward.

Presenting features

(a) Those due to failure of muscle relaxation. Masseter spasm after giving suxamethonium is associated with MH, but not all patients who get masseter spasm will go on to develop MH. When MH occurs a generalized increase of muscle tone develops during the anaesthetic even in the presence of adequate neuromuscular blockade. This is because the biochemical abnormality is intracellular and not mediated by the neuromuscular junction.

(b) Those due to hypermetabolism (which are often the first indication of the condition), which are:

1 Unexplained tachycardia.
2 Hypercarbia in the ventilated and hyperpnoea in the spontaneously breathing patient.
3 Cyanosis.
4 Dysrrhythmias, predominantly ventricular.
5 A rise in temperature.
6 Blood tests which show hypoxaemia, hyperkalaemia, hypercarbia, metabolic acidosis and hypocalcaemia.
7 Late events are myoglobinuria, acute renal and cardiac failure.

Management of the suspected or established case

Stop presenting the stimulus to the patient. Discontinue all volatile anaesthetics, change the breathing system and machine. Send for experienced help immediately and conclude surgery as soon as possible.

Treat the consequences of the hypermetabolism. Hyperventilate on 100% oxygen, give calcium and insulin/dextrose therapy for hyperkalaemia, sodium bicarbonate as determined by blood gases and appropriate drugs for persistent and haemodynamically detrimental dysrrhythmias.

Arrest the progress of the condition. Institute cooling measures commencing with surface cooling, progressing to viscus and body cavity irrigation and (in extreme cases) extracorporeal circulation as indicated. Give dantrolene (1 mg kg^{-1} every 5 minutes up to 10 mg kg^{-1}). Get an assistant to mix this because it is time consuming.

Maintain urine output at over 2 ml kg^{-1} min^{-1} with copious fluids, mannitol and frusemide to try and minimize the effects of myoglobinuria.

Once the acute episode has subsided, monitor the patient carefully on an ITU for the next 12–24 hours, commence oral dantrolene and continue close observation for 48–72 hours.

Do not forget to refer the patient to a centre for appropriate tests and genetic counselling.

Further reading

Denborough M. Malignant hyperthermia. *Lancet* 1998; 352: 1131–1136

Wappler F. Malignant hyperthermia. *Eur J Anaesthesiol* 2001; 18: 632–652

2   Summarize the aetiology, presentation and physiological consequences of aortic stenosis

Aetiology

Aortic stenosis presenting below the age of 60 years is usually rheumatic or congenital in origin. If a rheumatic origin, it is almost always accompanied by mitral valve disease. Calcified congenital bicuspid valve disease (commoner in men) presents from approximately 60 to 75 years. Degenerative calcification presents in patients over 70 years old and is commoner in women. Functional, but not pure, valvular stenosis at the supra-valvular and sub-valvular level are both very rare.

Presentation

There is usually a long latent period (typically 30 years) and the disease is well advanced at symptomatic presentation. Many patients have no symptoms and the condition is picked up incidentally (e.g. insurance or employment medicals). Symptoms are angina, dizziness, syncope on effort (low cardiac output), dyspnoea and the generalized presentation of left ventricular failure. Sudden death is not uncommon and some cases present with endocarditis. The ventricle becomes very dependent upon atrial contraction for adequate filling and a sudden deterioration in exercise tolerance or increased dyspnoea may be due to the onset of atrial fibrillation.

Physical signs are a small volume plateau pulse and a sustained and heaving apex beat (LVH). Auscultation reveals an ejection systolic murmur maximal in the second right intercostal space radiating to the neck, with a quiet delayed aortic second sound. There may be a thrill which radiates to the carotid arteries. The ECG shows LVH. The chest X-ray may be normal with a small-diameter aorta, which on occasions is dilated immediately distal to the aortic valve (post-stenotic dilatation). The aortic valve may be calcified. If there is just ventricular hypertrophy, the cardiopulmonary ratio will be preserved, but if LV dilatation has occurred the size of the heart shadow will be increased.

Physiological consequences

The progressive resistance to flow through the aortic valve causes the pressure in the left ventricle during systole to be higher in the left ventricle than in the aorta. The valve needs to be narrowed to about 25% of its normal area (which is approximately 3 cm^2) before there is a significant obstruction to flow across it. An area of 0.7 cm^2 is severe stenosis. The pressure drop across the valve can be calculated using Doppler as equal to four times the square of the blood velocity as measured in the ascending aorta. The clinical correlation with aortic gradients will vary but values of >50–90 mmHg are severe.

Over a long period stenosis of the valve orifice results in massive hypertrophy of the left ventricle, which becomes stiff and increasingly dependent upon the contribution from left atrial contraction for adequate ventricular filling. Ventricular dilatation occurs when there is associated regurgitation or when the ventricle fails. Angina may occur without significant coronary artery disease because of the precarious balance of oxygen supply and demand. The metabolic demands of the muscle are increased because of the high intraventricular wall pressures, and the thickness of the ventricular wall may itself hinder an adequate oxygen flux being transported from the distributing epicardial arteries to the subendocardial capillaries. Coronary filling is further impeded because the diseased valve distorts the aortic architecture and reduces the backflow of blood from the mainstream aortic flow into the coronary sinuses. The coronary ostia can also be narrowed by calcification. Optimum performance of the left ventricle becomes very dependent upon the correct heart rate. The rate must be low enough to allow adequate time for filling and ejection but not so slow that the end-diastolic volume is excessive.

Further reading

Goldstone JC, Pollard BJ. *Clinical Anaesthesia*. Churchill Livingstone, Edinburgh, 1996; 95–96, 517–519

3   Anaesthesia for magnetic resonance imaging (MRI)

A number of factors should be considered. These include:

1   Isolated environment.
2   Scan requirements.
3   Exclusion of ferromagnetic materials from scanner.
4   Limited patient access.
5   Limited recovery facilities.
6   Monitoring.

As with all anaesthesia in isolated areas, it is particularly important to check the anaesthetic equipment, drug cupboard, resuscitation equipment and layout of the room beforehand. Familiarize yourself with the staff in the unit and ensure that you have skilled assistance. If emergency help may be needed, call for it early, as it may be some time coming.

MRI scans usually take at least 15 minutes, with some lasting over an hour. During the scan, the patient must remain still; otherwise poor-quality pictures may result.

Ferromagnetic objects distort the magnetic field and degrade the picture quality. They may also pose a hazard within the magnetic field. A detailed check list should be completed prior to anaesthesia by both staff and patient to exclude the presence of ferromagnetic objects. As many pieces of anaesthetic equipment are ferromagnetic, these must be kept outside of the scanning room or securely bolted to the wall.

Anaesthesia is induced outside the MRI scanner. The anaesthetic machine and cylinders should be kept outside the 50-gauss line at all times. (Non-ferric anaesthetic machines have been manufactured.) As access to the patient during the scan is limited, a secure airway is essential. The patient is then transferred into the magnet area and positioned. Check that there is adequate length of breathing system and that an intravenous cannula is readily accessible with the patient in the magnet core. At the end of the procedure, the patient is removed from the scanner and transferred outside the 50-gauss line, before reversal of anaesthesia. The use of a suitable anaesthetic technique and the avoidance of heavy sedative premedication allow rapid recovery in the often limited recovery facilities.

Monitoring within the magnet core poses three problems. Firstly, metallic parts (metal connectors on non-invasive blood pressure (NIBP) devices, standard pulse oximeter probes) may degrade the picture quality. Secondly, the magnetic filed induces voltages in the blood flowing in the aorta, therefore degrading the ECG signal (leads V5 and V6 may be the least affected). Thirdly, loops of cable may get very hot and cause burns due to inductance from the magnetic field. Monitoring requires specialized ECG leads and non-metallic pulse oximeter and NIBP devices. Side-stream end-tidal CO_2 monitoring may be inaccurate with long sampling tubing, but is for useful monitoring CO_2 trends, disconnections and respiratory rate. It is usually not possible to watch the monitors and the patient at the same time. Ideally the anaesthetist observes the monitors (outside the scanner).

Further reading

Malviya S, Voepel-Lewis T, Eldevik OP, Rockwell DT, Wong JH, Tait AR. Sedation and general anaesthesia in children undergoing MRI and CT: adverse events and outcomes. *Br J Anaesth* 2000; 84(6): 743–748

4 Critical temperature, critical pressure, isotherms and triple point

The critical temperature is defined as the temperature above which a substance cannot be liquefied, however much the pressure is increased. The value for oxygen is −118.4°C, for nitrous oxide 36.4°C and for carbon dioxide 31°C.

The critical pressure is the pressure of a saturated vapour of the substance at its critical temperature. The value for oxygen is 50.8 bar, for nitrous oxide 72.5 bar and for carbon dioxide 73.8 bar.

Isotherms are lines on pressure–volume graphs which join together pressure volume combinations that exist at the same temperature. This is shown in figure below for nitrous oxide. Following the isotherm for 20°C from A to B represents the compression of the gaseous form of nitrous oxide. From B to C, as the volume is further reduced, with no increase in pressure, more of the gas phase condenses to a liquid, until at C it is all liquid. From C to D the pressure increases dramatically with a small decrease in volume because liquids are virtually incompressible. The isotherm at 36.4°C at a pressure of 72.5 bar just has a liquid saturated vapour point and is hence the critical temperature isotherm. The isotherm at 40°C is above the critical temperature and liquid never forms.

Close to the critical temperature, Boyle's law becomes inaccurate. Although the terms gas and vapour describe identical physical states, some authors refer to a gas as a vapour when it is below its critical temperature. This definition is followed in the figure.

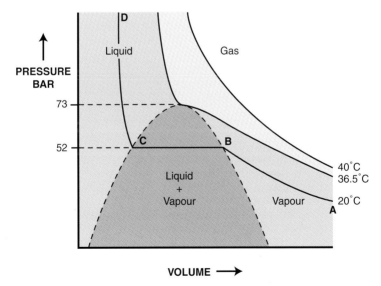

(After Parbrook, Davis and Parbrook, with permission from Butterworth Heinemann.)

The triple point is the point at which the gas, liquid and solid phases of a substance are in equilibrium. It occurs at a unique combination of temperature and pressure, which are $-218.8\,°C$ and 0.00152 bar for oxygen, $-90.7\,°C$ and 0.88 bar for nitrous oxide, and $-56.6\,°C$ and 5.17 bar for carbon dioxide.

5 Causes of lactic acidosis

Lactic acidosis may be divided into two types: those resulting from tissue hypoxia (type A) and those occurring in the absence of tissue hypoxia (type B). Type A is by far the more common cause. With modern monitoring techniques, a number of causes originally designated type B can be attributed to tissue hypoxia.

Type A

Evidence of tissue hypoxia:

- Shock (septic, cardiogenic, hypovolaemic).
- Regional ischaemia.
- Severe hypoxia.
- Severe anaemia.
- Carbon monoxide poisoning.
- Cyanide poisoning.
- Sepsis.
- Severe exercise.

Type B

B1 – presence of underlying disease:

- Diabetes mellitus.
- Liver disease.
- Malignancy.
- Phaeochromocytoma.

B2 – drugs and toxins:

- Biguanides – metformin.
- Alcohol, methanol, ethylene glycol.
- β_2-Adrenoceptor agonists.
- Paracetamol, salicylates.
- Fructose, sorbitol, xylitol.
- Antiretrovirals (nucleoside analogue reverse transcriptase inhibitors (NRTIs)), zidovudine.

B3 – inborn errors of metabolism:

- Glucose 6-phosphatase deficiency.
- Oxidative phosphorylation defects.
- Pyruvate dehydrogenase deficiency.

Further reading

Kirby DM, Crawford M, Cleary MA, Dahl HH, Dennett X, Thorburn DR. Respiratory chain complex I deficiency: an underdiagnosed energy generation disorder. *Neurology* 1999; 52(6): 1255–1564

Moyle G. Clinical manifestations and management of antiretroviral nucleoside analog-related mitochondrial toxicity. *Clin Ther* 2000; 22(8): 911–936

Parbrook GD, Davis PD, Parbrook EO. *Basic Physics and Measurement in Anaesthesia*. 3rd Edition. Butterworth Heinemann, Oxford, 1992

Vincent JL. Lactate levels in critically ill patients. *Acta Anaesthesiol Scand Suppl* 1995; 107261–107266

6   The functional residual capacity (FRC)

Definition

The FRC is the remaining lung volume at the end of a relaxed expiration – the point when the natural tendency of the lungs to collapse is exactly balanced by the chest wall recoil. It is the sum of two volumes: the residual volume and the expiratory reserve volume.

Magnitude

In the average adult the FRC is approximately 2.5–3 litres in the upright position. It increases with height, decreases with obesity and is slightly lower in females.

Factors affecting the FRC

The FRC changes with posture, being greatest in the upright position and reduced by approximately 25% when supine. It is increased in obstructive respiratory disorders and decreased in restrictive lung disease. Both CPAP and PEEP increase FRC, the volume change being related to the product of the compliance and pressure change.

Relevance to anaesthesia

The FRC is a respiratory gas buffer zone, preventing breath-to-breath swings in PaO_2. After adequate pre-oxygenation, it is the oxygen store which will be utilized during any subsequent period of apnoea. The FRC is reduced after the induction of anaesthesia by around 15–20% regardless of the mode of ventilation. The cause is thought to be principally a reduction in inspiratory muscle tone. After major abdominal or thoracic surgery it remains reduced and may increase the episodes of postoperative desaturation, atelectasis and chest infection.

Measurement

1   The laboratory standard is body plethysmography, first used clinically by DuBois et al. in the 1950s. The subject is enclosed in an airtight chamber. At the end of a normal expiration, a shutter occludes the mouthpiece and the subject attempts to expand his lungs by a series of panting breaths. The resultant pressure changes within the chamber can be related to lung volume by the application of Boyle's law. This method measures all gas, including that trapped behind closed airways.

2   The nitrogen washout method was introduced by Darling et al. in 1940. In this the subject breaths 100% oxygen for several minutes and the expired gas is collected and analysed for nitrogen. This nitrogen was originally in the FRC at a concentration around 79%, hence FRC can be derived.

3   Helium dilution: this is usually based on a closed circuit equilibration method described by Meneely and Kaltrieder in 1949. At end expiration the subject is connected to a system with a known volume and known concentration of the inert gas helium ($He^{[1]}$). The subject then breathes (or is ventilated) quietly until a new steady state is reached and the new lower concentration of helium (diluted by the FRC) is noted ($He^{[2]}$). During the procedure carbon dioxide is usually absorbed by soda lime and oxygen consumption is replaced. Helium is a very insoluble gas and uptake into the body is negligible and can be ignored over the time course of the measurement. The FRC may be calculated from the following:

$$He^{[1]} \times \text{circuit volume} = He^{[2]} \times (\text{circuit volume} + FRC)$$

Further reading

Nunn JF. *Applied Respiratory Physiology*, 4th edition. Butterworth Heinemann, Oxford, 1993

---

7   **Endothelial derived relaxant factor (EDRF) – NO**

In 1980, it was demonstrated that the vascular relaxation induced by acetylcholine (ACh) was dependent upon the presence of an intact vascular endothelium and that a labile humoral compound, later called endothelium derived relaxation factor (EDRF), was responsible for this phenomenon. There are also constricting factors: EDCF. Subsequent investigation revealed that endothelium-dependent relaxation was present in a wide variety of vascular tissues including artery, vein and the micro-circulation. Numerous chemical signals were shown to cause this phenomenon, including ACh, adenine nucleotides, thrombin, substance P and bradykinin. Physical stimuli such as hypoxia, increase in blood flow and electrical stimulation also invoked the response. In contrast, it has been demonstrated that another distinct set of endogenous and exogenous substances, including nitro-vasodilators, atrial natriuretic factor, β-adrenergic agonists and prostacyclin, do not require the local presence of endothelium and EDRF to cause vascular relaxation.

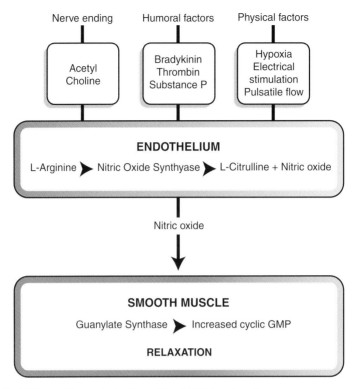

(After Wilkes, with permission from Churchill Livingstone.)

Further studies reported that EDRF was a very short-lived substance with a physiological half-life of only seconds and that endothelial tissue also produced a basal release of EDRF in the absence of ACh stimulation. EDRF was also shown to inhibit platelet aggregation and this action was synergistic with the similar property of prostacyclin. Most importantly it was shown that the action of EDRF on cells was to directly increase intracellular cyclic GMP levels. Subsequently EDRF was characterized as the gas nitric oxide (NO). An enzyme system, nitric oxide synthase, was described which utilized the amino acid L-arginine as a substrate, NADPH as a cofactor and L-citrulline and NO as products. Production of NO is modulated in endothelium by both chemical and physical stimuli and acts directly upon underlying smooth muscle cGMP.

NO has been described as the 'endogenous vasodilator' and its discovery has questioned the conventional physiological picture of a vascular tree with a tone globally controlled by the autonomic nervous system and relaxed locally by products of cellular respiration. It has been postulated that the vascular tree is kept in a continual state of vasodilatation by local EDRF release, and organ blood flow autoregulation is thus directly controlled by physical and chemical stimulation of vascular endothelium. NO-produced vasodilatation occurs locally and represents a simple, elegant, self-regulating control system for local organ blood flow.

The discovery of NO also helps describe the actions of the nitro-vasodilators. Glyceryl trinitrate is humorally degraded to NO through a non-enzymatic reaction with cysteine and sodium nitroprusside which spontaneously releases NO in solution. The identification of a simple molecule as a potent biological transmitter and effector substance has changed the current views of many areas of research. The L-arginine:NO pathway has been discovered in many diverse biological areas outside the scope of this discussion. It represents the transducer mechanism for soluble guanylate synthase and is thus a central mechanism by which cells regulate their function and communicate with other cell groups. The understanding of the physiology of the cardiovascular system has been fundamentally altered by this research and a mechanism by which blood vessels can locally regulate their tone has been demonstrated.

An imbalance between EDCF and EDRF, termed 'pulmonary endothelial dysfunction', may contribute aspects of pulmonary disease, in particular in hypoxia-induced pulmonary hypertension.

Further reading

Chen YF, Oparil S. Endothelial dysfunction in the pulmonary vascular bed. *Am J Med Sci* 2000; 320(4): 223–232

Ignaro LJ, Cirino G, Casini A, Napoli C. Nitric oxide as a signaling molecule in the vascular system: an overview. *J Cardiovasc Pharmacol* 1999; 34(6): 879–886

Moncada S, Palmer RMJ, Higgs EA. Nitric oxide: physiology, pathophysiology and pharmacology. *Pharmacol Rev* 1991; 43: 109–141

Wilkes MP. Endothelial derived relaxant factor. *Curr Anaesth Crit Care* 1996; 7: 52–60

8   Anaesthetic problems in acromegaly

Acromegaly is characterized by overgrowth of bone, connective tissue and viscera due to prolonged excessive release of growth hormone. There is enlargement of the heart, liver and thyroid. If treated, the patient will be on hormone replacement therapy. It is an important condition for the anaesthetist for a number of reasons:

* Difficult airway management.
* Hypertension.
* Cardiac failure (sometimes secondary to a cardiomyopathy).
* Sleep apnoea.
* Diabetes.

Local or regional anaesthesia should be considered as alternatives, but even if chosen, difficult airway management needs to be anticipated in case there are problems with toxicity or sedation. These patients have large lips, jaw, tongue and epiglottis. Hypertrophy of the pharyngeal and laryngeal structures may make the anatomy difficult to interpret, the cords may not be seen and the larynx may be resistant to external manipulation. Management of the airway on a face mask is likely to be difficult and suitable for only short operations. Care is required with nasopharyngeal airways because the hypertrophied nasal mucosa can make passage difficult and haemorrhage is easy to provoke. There are no published reports of the use of the laryngeal mask airway in acromegalics.

If intubation is required, the best technique depends upon the individual patient and anaesthetist. Skilled, fibre-optic awake intubation is probably the safest course of action, but may be unpalatable to the patient and unnecessary in many cases. Although theoretically correct, deepening anaesthesia with volatile agents and assessing the larynx before attempting intubation is likely to be difficult to do smoothly. If the intubation on preoperative assessment or from a previous anaesthetic record appears relatively straightforward, pre-oxygenation, i.v. induction and a short-acting relaxant is probably the sequence of choice. A long-bladed laryngoscope and introducers can be useful. Have available uncut endotracheal tubes of less than the anticipated diameter: they may be needed if there is supra- or subglottic stenosis. All the normal equipment and facilities for managing difficult intubation need to be available. Although there are no specific reports of it in the literature, acromegalics would seem likely to be a group at risk of postoperative hypoxia.

Further reading

Chan VWS, Tindall S. Anaesthesia for Transsphenoidal Surgery in a Patient with Extreme Giantism. *Br J Anaesth* 1998; 60: 464–468

Hakala P, Randell T, Valli H. Laryngoscopy and fibreoptic intubation in acromegalic patients. *Br J Anaesth* 1998; 80(3): 345–347

Hutton P, Cooper GM. *Guidelines in Clinical Anaesthesia*. Blackwell Scientific, Oxford, 1985: 223–225

Seidman PA, Kofke WA, Policare R, Young M. Anaesthetic complications of acromegaliy. *Br J Anaesth* 2000; 84(2): 179–782

9 Suxamethonium apnoea

Suxamethonium apnoea is the commonly used term to describe prolonged paralysis following the normal therapeutic dose of suxamethonium. The transient effects of a single dose of suxamethonium are due to its rapid hydrolysis by plasma cholinesterase (pseudocholinesterase). This occurs in two stages: initially, choline groups are removed to produce succinyl monocholine, which is itself further broken down to form succinic acid and choline. Prolongation of the effect of suxamethonium is caused by the failure of breakdown, which may be due to decreased availability, inhibition or genetic polymorphism of the patient's pseudocholinesterase.

Decreased availability

Plasma cholinesterase is synthesized by the liver and severe hepatic dysfunction (usually accompanied by marked hypoalbuminaemia) can prolong its effect. Cholinesterase levels are also reduced:

- In pregnancy.
- In the malnourished.
- Following plasmapheresis.

Enzyme inhibition or competing substrates

Drugs which inhibit plasma cholinesterase extend the action of suxamethonium and some, e.g. tetrahydroaminocrine ('tacrine'), have been used therapeutically for this purpose. Other drugs which affect its breakdown include ecthiopate, edrophonium, neostigmine, cyclophosphamide, organophosphorus compounds, trimetaphan and alkylating agents.

Genetic polymorphism

This is caused by inherited atypical plasma cholinesterase. Four allomorphic genes have been identified at a single locus of chromosome 3. These genes are called E_1^u, E_1^a, E_1^f and E_1^s; respectively, and produce the normal enzyme, the atypical enzyme, the fluoride-resistant enzyme and the absent (silent) enzyme. The different combinations of these genes give classical genotypes as shown in the table below. The commonest genetic variant (the atypical enzyme) can be distinguished from the normal enzyme by its resistance to inhibition by the local anaesthetic chincocaine (dibucaine). The 'dibucaine number' is defined as the percentage enzyme inhibition produced by 10^{-5} M dibucaine, using benzoylcholine as the substrate. In recent years, using DNA cloning techniques, at least six further allomorphic genes have been identified and another distinct locus may be responsible for increased cholinesterase activity.

The common classical genetic variants of plasma cholinesterase

Phenotype	Frequency (%)	P Chincocaine activity (U l^{-1})	Dibucaine number
E^uE^u	95–97	690–1560	79–87
E^uE^a	2–4	320–1150	55–72
E^aE^a	0.04	140–730	14–27

Further reading

Calvey TN, Williams NE. *Principles and Practice of Pharmacology for Anaesthetists*, 2nd edition. Blackwell Scientific, Oxford, 1991: 276–277

10 | Damage to the brachial plexus under general anaesthesia

Under anaesthesia, damage occurs by a combination of traction and compression in the following ways:

1 During surgery on the axilla, unintentional positioning or leaning by the surgeon and/or his/her assistant, the arm may be forcibly abducted and externally rotated. This stretches the cords across the glenoid head and the trunks are compressed in the reduced space between the clavicle and first rib. The action is intensified if the weight of the patient prevents rotation of the scapula, contributing to abduction of the arm, and if the arm is insufficiently supported and drops away posteriorly from the side of the body.

2 By similar mechanisms to the above, with the hands above the head in a supine patient, abduction puts the plexus at risk.

3 Lateral operating positions with the arm suspended on a badly positioned bar can cause effects similar to the above.

4 When the patient is in the Trendelenburg position, wristlets may pull on the upper arms and stretch the upper plexus, and shoulder braces may compress the plexus between the clavicle and first rib (if placed medially) or drag it downwards (if placed laterally).

5 Neck extension with lateral flexion stretches the contralateral plexus (the head needs supporting in the lateral position).

6 Sternotomy and rib retraction stretch the lower plexus.

Diagnosis is by clinical examination and electromyographic studies. It is essential to distinguish plexus injuries from those of peripheral nerves. Electromyography enables the extent and level of damage to be quantified and in addition, by stimulating electrically, allows an assessment of prognosis.

Recovery is usually good. In general, sensory function recovers faster than motor, and muscles innervated by lower cervical roots tend to recover before those supplied by the upper roots.

Prevention is by careful positioning, support and padding of the patient to prevent the abnormal postures described above.

Further reading

Ben-David B, Stahl S. Prognosis of intraoperative brachial plexus injury: a review of 22 cases. *Br J Anaesth* 1997; 79(4): 440–445

Payan J. Nerve injury. In: Taylor TH, Major E (eds). *Hazards and Complications of Anaesthesia*, 2nd edition. Churchill Livingstone, Edinburgh, 1993: 561–517

11 | The renin–angiotensin system

The renin–angiotensin system is involved in the control of blood pressure and fluid balance. Renin is a glycoprotein (MW 37 326), formed from two pre-hormones (pro-renin and pre-pro-renin), which is synthesized in and secreted from the juxtaglomerular apparatus of the renal tubule. The half-life of renin is approximately 80 minutes. Its secretion increases in hypovolaemia, cardiac failure, cirrhosis and renal artery stenosis: it decreases by the action of angiotensin II and vasopressin (antidiuretic hormone).

Renin acts upon the circulating glycoprotein angiotensinogen to produce angiotensin I (a non-active precursor), II and III. The conversion of angiotensin I to II is dependent upon angiotensin-converting enzyme (ACE) and this enzyme is disabled by the ACE inhibitor group of antihypertensive drugs. Angiotensin II is a powerful vasoconstrictor with a half-life of a few minutes which causes aldosterone release from the adrenal cortex and noradrenaline release from sympathetic nerve endings. It also stimulates thirst and the release of vasopressin and acts directly on renal tubules to retain salt and water. It also may have other effects and it has been suggested that the renin–angiotensin system influences the fibrinolytic system so that pharmacological interventions that reduce the activity of angiotensin II may have favourable effects on fibrinolytic balance in the context of adverse cardiovascular events.

Pharmacological interruption of the renin–angiotensin system is possible at three major sites: the ACE, the AT1 receptor and at the interaction of renin with its substrate, angiotensinogen.

Further reading

Mazze RI. Renal physiology. In: Miller RD (ed.). *Anaesthesia*, 3rd edition. Churchill Livingstone, Edinburgh, 1994: 630–606

Mirendon JV, Grissom TE. Anesthetic implications of the renin–angiotensin system and angiotensin-converting enzyme inhibitors. *Anesth Analg* 1991; 72: 667–673

Vaughan DE. Angiotensin, fibrinolysis, and vascular homeostasis. *Am J Cardiol* 2001; 87(8A): 18C–24C

12 | **Pulmonary barotrauma**

Pulmonary barotrauma (PBT) is lung damage secondary to excessive airways pressure or to excessive shear forces in the airways. It manifests itself as pneumothorax, pneumomediastinum, pneumoperitoneum or subcutaneous emphysema resulting from passage of air from the tracheobronchial tree and alveoli through tissue planes. The maximum danger of its occurrence is the combination of diseased or stiff lungs (long-standing chronic obstructive airways disease, acute asthma, respiratory distress syndrome, adult respiratory distress syndrome), with high inspiratory pressures and volumes (which may be necessary for adequate oxygenation).

It is particularly associated with

- High levels of PEEP.
- High inspiratory flows.

- Excessive tidal volumes.
- Rapid rate of change of volume.

There is the suggestion that part of the mechanism of barotrauma is the production of inflammatory mediators in response to mechanical injury to the lung but this is still under investigation.

The most feared and potentially life-threatening complication is a tension pneumothorax developing unrecognized during IPPV. The impact of this pressurized extra-alveolar air on pulmonary and cardiovascular function can be devastating. If suspected clinically with the appropriate accompanying physical signs, relief should be undertaken immediately by insertion of a large-bore i.v. cannula (going just above a rib to avoid the neurovascular bundle). If, however, the pneumothorax is suspected clinically early in its development and time is available for evaluation, a portable chest radiograph should be taken to confirm diagnosis and aid chest tube placement. Under these non-emergency conditions, insertion of a chest tube in the fifth intercostal space in the mid-axillary line avoids the latissimus dorsi and pectoralis major muscles and allows the tube to be easily directed to the superior intrapleural space. In some cases evidence of pulmonary interstitial emphysema may be seen on the chest X-ray (perivascular air, hilar air streaks, subpleural bullae), before the development of a severe pneumothorax.

Subcutaneous emphysema results from mediastinal air tracking through the tissue planes and in some cases can completely obscure the normal anatomy of the neck, making neck line placement not only impossible but the attempts to do so potentially dangerous. Previous neck surgery or pleural scarring may, in rare cases, prevent the mediastinal decompression. Pneumopericardium, which is also rare, presents like tamponade and is drained using the same technique as for a pericardial effusion. If pneumoperitoneum is causing unacceptable pressurized distension of the abdomen, it can be decompressed by the placement of a peritoneal dialysis catheter.

Barotrauma is best prevented rather than managed. Decreasing the risk of barotrauma is done by:

1 Minimizing the number of mechanically delivered breaths (in both neonates and adults).
2 Minimizing peak inspiratory pressures by appropriate adjustment of flow rates, volumes, sedation, analgesia and relaxants. This may require PEEP to minimize shear forces.
3 Maintaining the intravascular volume.
4 Using selective (independent) lung ventilation in cases of unilateral malfunction.

It must be remembered that a respiratory death should not be allowed to occur in one's efforts to prevent barotrauma: the factors necessary to allow adequate gas exchange and oxygen delivery should, however, be adjusted so as to minimize the chance of its occurrence.

Further reading

Gammon RB, Shin MS, Groves RH, Hardin JM, Hsu C, Buchalter SE. Clinical risk factors for pulmonary barotrauma: a multivariate analysis. *Am J Respir Crit Care Me*d 1995; 152(4 Pt 1): 1235–1240

Gillette MA, Hess DR. Ventilator-induced lung injury and the evolution of lung-protective strategies in acute respiratory distress syndrome. *Respir Care* 2001; 46(2): 130–148

Kirby RR, Taylor RW, Civetta JM. Pulmonary barotrauma. In: *A Pocket Compendium of Critical Care: Immediate Concerns*. Lippincott, Philadelphia, 1990: 376–383

Paper Two Write short notes on the following topics. Do not miss out any questions and remember that there are only 3 hours in total to complete this paper.

1 Anaesthesia in patients fitted with a pacemaker
2 Control of intracranial pressure
3 Positive end-expiratory pressure
4 Coaxial breathing systems
5 The anaesthetic management of patients with thyroid disease
6 Monoamine oxidase inhibitors
7 Sickle cell disease
8 The anaesthetic implications of severe obesity
9 Anaesthesia in a patient with myasthenia gravis
10 Post-herpetic neuralgia
11 Pudendal nerve block
12 PHi (gastric tonometry)

1 Anaesthesia in patients fitted with a pacemaker

Most patients carry a European pacemaker registration card that contains information about the pacemaker type, reason for its implant, place where it was implanted and lead type (unipolar or bipolar). While many pacemakers inserted are on-demand ventricular pacing units (VVI), a significant number of new pacemakers are atrial ventricular pacing units (DDD). If possible, the pacemaker should be checked by a pacing technician before anaesthesia.

Preoperative assessment is important as coexisting disease is common: 50% have ischaemic heart disease, 20% are hypertensive and 10% are diabetic, and many will be on a variety of drugs, some with cardiac actions. A recurrence of symptoms, such as dizziness or syncope, may indicate pacemaker malfunction. An electrocardiogram (ECG), chest X-ray and electrolytes should be checked. Surgical diathermy may affect pacemakers in three ways:

1 It may lead to inhibition of the unit, resulting in no output and potentially asystole.

2 It may induce eddy currents in the pacing lead, resulting in ventricular arrhythmias including ventricular fibrillation.

3 The software programming in some DDD units may be erased by the diathermy, resulting in potentially unsuitable pacing parameters.

If diathermy is essential, it should be used in short bursts if possible. Bipolar is preferable to unipolar. If unipolar diathermy is essential, the diathermy plate should be sited well away from the heart and pacemaker, such as on the thigh. If unipolar diathermy is to be used, the pacemaker should ideally be put into asynchronous mode (VOO or DOO) preoperatively. If the ECG monitor is unable to reject the interference from diathermy, it is essential that the patient's pulse is felt when the ECG cannot be interpreted.

Full monitoring is essential before induction of anaesthesia. A large magnet must be easily available. Before using the magnet 'in anger', it must be established that the magnet will convert the pacemaker into asynchronous mode, as some DD units do not go into DOO mode when a magnet is applied to them and may be reprogrammed if diathermy and a magnet are used simultaneously. A defibrillator must be available, ideally with the capacity for external transcutaneous pacing. In the emergency situation, particularly when there is doubt about the pacemaker type or its reliability, the pacing paddles should be put on before induction of anaesthesia. In addition, an isoprenaline infusion should be available.

Prevention of hypoxia is essential, not only because many patients have ischaemic heart disease, but also because hypoxia may lead to either loss of pacemaker capture and possibly asystole, or loss of sensing, leading to inadvertent pacing and potentially serious arrhythmias. Patients should therefore be pre-oxygenated. A cardiostable induction is essential, as many patients are unable to mount a compensatory tachycardia in response to vasodilatation, which may lead to severe hypotension. Suxamethonium is not contraindicated, but the muscle fasciculations may result in transient pacemaker inhibition (VVI and DDD) or inappropriate stimulation (DDD).

Volatile anaesthesia agents increase the pacing threshold, potentially leading to loss of capture, though this is generally not a problem. A technique of IPPV with a relaxant, N_2O, O_2, opioid and volatile agent should be used for all but the shortest of cases. Postoperatively, the patient should be monitored until fully recovered and the pacemaker is shown to be functioning correctly.

Further reading

Bourke ME. The patient with a pacemaker or related device. *Can J Anaesth* 1996; 43(5 Pt 2): R24–R41

Deroy R, Graham TR. Pacemaker and anaesthesia. *Curr Anaesth Crit Care* 1995; 6: 171–179

Pacemaker codes. NASPE/BPEG

Position	I	II	III	IV	V
Category	Chamber(s) paced	Chamber(s) sensed	Response to sensing	Programmability, rate modulation	Anti-tachyarrhythmia functions
	0 = None A = Atrium	0 = None A = Atrium	0 = None T = Triggered	0 = None P = Simple programmable M = Multi-programmable	0 = None P = Pacing (anti-arrhythmic)
	V = Ventricle D = Dual (A+V)	V = Ventricle D = Dual (A+V)	I = Inhibited D = Dual (T+I)	R = Rate modulation	S = Shock D = Dual (P+S)

This is a code to represent types of pacemaker. The first three letters each designate an antibradycardic function while the last two, often absent, represent other functions such as sophisticated programming, 'R' rate modulation or defibrillator function, 'S' shock. So VAT would be ventricle paced but senses the atrium and uses that to trigger ventricular pacing.

2 Control of intracranial pressure

The skull is a rigid box containing the brain, cerebrospinal fluid (CSF) and blood. Changes in the volume of any of the contents may affect intracranial pressure (ICP). As the volume of one constituent changes, a compensatory change occurs in the others to keep ICP constant. When compensatory mechanisms are no longer sufficient, the compliance of the intracranial cavity is greatly reduced and the ICP rises.

The normal level of ICP is 7–10 mmHg. Increasing ICP affects cerebral perfusion pressure (CCP) as CPP = MAP – ICP, resulting in focal ischaemia. Further

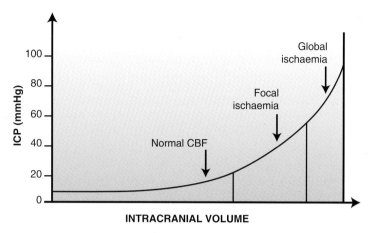

(After Dodds, with permission from Churchill Livingstone.)

increases lead to displacement of intracranial contents, brain herniation and global ischaemia. Control of ICP is aimed at reducing intracranial volume while maintaining adequate cerebral perfusion, and should ideally be guided by monitoring of the ICP. Methods of controlling the ICP include:

1 Prevention of hypoxia and hypotension.
2 Treatment of underlying cause where possible, for example, surgical removal of haematoma.
3 Avoidance of factors that may raise ICP, which include:
   (a) Cerebral vasodilation from hypoxia, hypercarbia and certain anaesthetic agents such as halothane, enflurane and ketamine.
   (b) Vascular engorgement from neck flexion and rotation, positive end-expiratory pressure, coughing and volume overload.
4 Specific treatment for raised ICP:
   (a) Head-up tilt. This aids venous drainage from the head. A tilt of up to 30° will reduce ICP but maintain CPP.
   (b) Controlled hyperventilation. Lowering $PaCO_2$ to 3.5–4.0 kPa results in cerebro-vasoconstriction and decreased cerebral blood volume. The effect is immediate, but lasts only few hours. Excess vasoconstriction may worsen cerebral ischaemia.
   (c) Diuretics. Osmotic diuretics, such as mannitol, establish an osmotic gradient across the capillary wall which draws fluid from the extracellular space. Excessive use may lead to increased interstitial osmolality and worsen brain oedema. Their onset of action is between 15 and 60 minutes. Loop diuretics, such as frusemide, increase plasma osmolality by diuresis and reduce CSF formation directly. They have a slower onset of action, but do not raise intravascular volume. They appear to act synergistically with osmotic diuretics.

(d) Hypnotic agents. Drugs such as barbiturates and propofol lower ICP by decreasing cerebral metabolic rate and so cerebral blood flow. They may cause hypotension and so reduce CPP. Inotropes may be necessary to maintain CPP at about 70 mmHg.

(e) Steroids. These are useful in reducing cerebral oedema associated with tumours, but are associated with higher morbidity and mortality when used in head injury.

(f) CSF drainage. This may be performed through a ventricular catheter.

(g) Severe fluid restriction is now rarely used to decrease ICP. It may worsen cerebral ischaemia and may also cause hypernatraemia and renal failure.

Further reading

Dodds C. Control of intracranial pressure. *Curr Anaesth Crit Care* 1997; 8: 91–96

Marik P, Chen K, Varon J, Fromm R, Stembach GL. Management of increased intracranial pressure: a review for clinicians. *J Emerg Med* 1999; 17(4): 711–719

North B, Reilly P. Measurement and manipulation of intracranial pressure. *Curr Anaesth Crit Care* 1994; 5: 23–28

---

3 Positive end-expiratory pressure

Positive end-expiratory pressure (PEEP) is the application of positive airways pressure throughout expiration. Devices for administering PEEP include:

1 Electronically controlled expiratory valve, which is activated when the expiratory pressure reaches a given value.

2 Spring-loaded disc valve, where an adjustable spring provides tension against a disc resting on the exhalation port. Spring tension is varied by a threaded screw.

3 Water-weighted diaphragm, where water is separated by a flexible diaphragm seated on the exhalation port. The height of the water column regulates the PEEP value.

The beneficial pulmonary affects of PEEP are:

• Increased functional residual capacity (FRC): The presence of PEEP may prevent alveoli collapsing. At levels of 10 cmH$_2$O or less, PEEP is responsible for increasing the volume of patent alveoli.

• Recruitment: above 10 cmH$_2$O collapsed alveoli may be recruited. This increases the surface area available for gas exchange and improves V/Q mismatch, so improving oxygenation.

• Redistribution of lung water: PEEP does not reduce extravascular water in the lungs but facilitates its movement away from areas of gas exchange, so improving oxygen diffusion into the alveolar capillary.

The pulmonary adverse affects of PEEP are:

- Increased dead space ventilation. This occurs particularly in lungs with non-uniform pathology where normal alveoli can be over-distended, compressing surrounding capillaries and so diminishing their blood supply.
- Barotrauma.

PEEP also affects other systems:

- Cardiovascular system. Cardiac output is reduced as increased intrathoracic pressure leads to a reduction in venous return and so reduced preload. Right ventricular afterload increases because of compression of pulmonary vasculature. PEEP may result in an overall reduction in oxygen delivery if the reduction in cardiac output is greater than the increase in arterial oxygen content. Fluid administration and inotropes may be needed to counteract this.
- Kidneys. Renal perfusion pressure is reduced owing to reduced venous return and reduced cardiac output, which results in a reduced glomerular filtration rate and decreased urine output. Activation of the renin–angiotensin system and increased levels of antidiuretic hormone lead to increased water retention. Total lung water may increase as a result.
- Central nervous system. Increased intrathoracic pressure may impede venous return from the head. This can lead to an increase in intracranial pressure if intracranial compliance is low.

The clinically appropriate level of PEEP is the least amount that will achieve adequate arterial oxygenation at a satisfactory FiO_2 without significant impairment of tissue perfusion.

The indications for PEEP are:

1. Acute lung injury/acute respiratory disease.
2. Intubated patients. FRC is reduced in intubated patients. Part of this may be due to bypassing the sphincter function of the glottis. Low levels of PEEP may help by substituting for glottis function.
3. Post cardiac surgery. PEEP may help reduce bleeding after surgery through tamponading bleeding sites.
4. Cardiac failure. PEEP improves oxygenation but does not reduce lung water.

Further reading

Fessler HE. Heart–lung interactions: applications in the critically ill. *Eur Respir J* 1997; 10(1): 226–237

Hawker FF. PEEP and CPAP. *Curr Anaesth Crit Care* 1996; 7: 236–242

Lu Q, Rouby JJ. Measurement of pressure–volume curves in patients on mechanical ventilation: methods and significance. *Crit Care* 2000; 4(2): 91–100

4 Coaxial breathing systems

Coaxial breathing systems are those where the outer corrugated hose contains a smaller-diameter tube so that gas moves in either direction within the whole system. The two coaxial systems in present use are the Lack (Mapleson A) and Bain (Mapleson D) circuits.

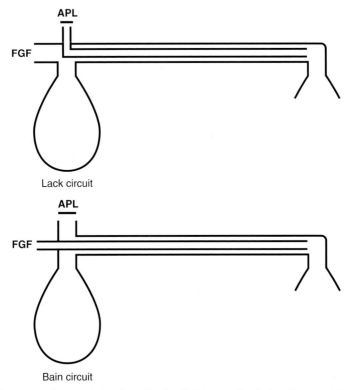

(After Lack, with permission from Blackwell Science; after Bain, with permission from Canadian Anaesthesiologists' Society.)

Lack circuit

This was first described in 1976 and was an attempt to improve on the convenience of the Magill circuit and reduce theatre pollution. In the Magill circuit the expiratory spill valve is sited as close to the patient as possible. This makes it liable to be covered by surgical drapes and adds weight to the face mask or endotracheal tube. In the Lack arrangement the outer tube carries fresh gas and the inner tube carries expired gas and is connected to the expiratory spill valve at the anaesthetic machine end of the system. The advantages of this circuit are that the spill valve is accessible and attachment of scavenging systems is facilitated. The physics of the system ensure a relatively low resistance. During expiration, as expired gas flows back towards the reservoir bag it is met by the fresh gas inflow, the pressure rises and flow is diverted towards the expiratory valve. If the flow is adequate no expired gas reaches the reservoir bag, so no mixing occurs.

The inner tube has to be of adequate diameter to prevent too high a resistance to flow in expiration. The outer tube must be of sufficient diameter to prevent too high a resistance to flow in inspiration and the outer tube must be of sufficient volume to prevent expired gas reaching the reservoir. The fresh gas requirements are equivalent to those of the conventional Mapleson A and so it is an efficient circuit for spontaneous ventilation.

The main disadvantage of the coaxial arrangement is that of disconnection of the inner tube, results in reduced efficiency in removing carbon dioxide. The outer tube is partially transparent so that the inner tube can be viewed.

Bain circuit

This is a modification of the Mapleson D circuit first described in 1972. Fresh gas flows through a narrow inner tube and is delivered to the patient end of the system. Expired gas passes down the outer corrugated tube and is vented through the expiratory valve near the reservoir bag sited at the machine end. Fresh gas flows necessary to prevent rebreathing are similar to those of the Mapleson D. It is efficient when used for controlled ventilation where flows of 70 ml kg^{-1} min^{-1} will produce normocarbia. Recommended fresh gas flows for spontaneous ventilation are 200–300 ml kg^{-1} min^{-1}. It is a lightweight and convenient circuit and scavenging is possible from the expiratory spill valve.

As with the Lack circuit, the major disadvantage is that of possible disconnection of the inner tube. This results in greatly increased dead space and hypercarbia. The outer tube must be transparent to enable viewing of the inner tube.

Testing. Occlude the inner tube and test for rapid pressure rise and valve opening at the machine. Occlude outer tube and watch bag fill. Inner tube integrity may then be assessed using the Pethick test, where the reservoir bag is filled while the patient end of the circuit is occluded. The patient end is then opened and oxygen flushed through. If the inner tube is intact a Venturi effect results in emptying of the reservoir bag.

Further reading

Bain JA, Spoerel WE. A streamlined anaesthetic system. *Can J Anaesth* 1972; 19: 426–435

Lack JA. Theatre pollution control. *Anaesthesia* 1976; 31: 259–262

5 The anaesthetic management of patients with thyroid disease

Thyrotrophin-releasing factor from the hypothalamus causes the release of thyroid-stimulating factor by the anterior pituitary, which increases release of T_3 and T_4. Hyperthyroidism is due to the overproduction of T_3 or T_4 by the thyroid, usually in conjunction with undetectable levels of thyroid-stimulating hormone.

Hyperthyroidism should ideally be treated prior to surgery to make the patient euthyroid, but the treated hyperthyroid patient can still have 'thyroid storms' postoperatively. The commonly used drugs can cause immunological suppression and there is a strong association with other autoimmune disorders. Awareness of the other organs implicated in the multiple endocrine adenoma (MEA) syndromes is important.

Preoperative assessment should look for the classic symptoms and signs. In particular, tachycardia and tremor might indicate inadequate control. Assessment of the trachea is vital, as is pre- and postoperative vocal cord inspection. Computed tomography will demonstrate mediastinal compression or invasion.

Anaesthetic technique varies, but isoflurane is currently the volatile agent of choice as it has the least effect on T_4 levels. Intubation may be difficult, especially if there is an enlarged tongue. Armoured endotracheal tubes have been advocated by some authorities. Damage to the recurrent laryngeal nerve may occur and it is on this basis that the some clinicians only extubate after confirmation of bilateral vocal cord movement. This is technically difficult, may complicate extubation itself and is not always informative. Following extubation reintubation may be necessary if there is stridor of any kind. This may be due to nerve injury, tracheal oedema, formation of a peritracheal haematoma or there may be tracheomalacia from pressure damage. Superior laryngeal nerve damage may result in aspiration due to lack of sensation around the piriform fossa.

Thyroid storm. This occurs in untreated or partially treated patients and can be triggered by infection. There is often a combination of fever, tachycardia, cardiac failure and loss of consciousness. Treatment involves resuscitation, β-blockade and sodium iodide treatment.

Hypothyroidism and hypoparathyroidism can both occur following thyroid resection and may be very acute.

Further reading

Farling PA. Thyroid disease. *Br J Anaesth* 2000; 85(1): 15–28

6 Monoamine oxidase inhibitors

There are two common monoamine oxidase enzyme systems: MAO-A is found in the CNS and MAO-B is found in the liver, lungs and kidneys. The more modern inhibitors of these enzymes are much more specific than the original drugs and often have a much shorter elimination half-life. They have predictable actions: they reduce sympathetic tone, the stress response and can cause postural hypotension. Hypoglycaemia may occur because of a synergy with insulin. Monoamine oxidase inhibitors often increase the patient's sensitivity to the sedative effects of anaesthetic drugs and benzodiazepines. They can decrease plasma cholinesterase levels and prolong the action of suxamethonium and mivacurium. Pethidine is absolutely contraindicated because of hyperexcitation (hypertension, pyrexia, coma, tachycardia and convulsions); morphine is the safest opiate to use. Remifentanil is reported as safe.

Unless the drug is named, it has to be assumed that the older generation of drug is being used. Unless an emergency occurs, all surgery should be delayed for 2 weeks to allow regeneration of monoamine oxidase. The postural hypotension limits the value of regional anaesthesia and i.v. agents should be used with extreme caution. Rebound vasoconstriction occurs with the use of vasopressors, causing profound hypertension. Treatment of the hypertensive crises may require nitroprusside infusions and invasive monitoring is advisable perioperatively.

Further reading

Smith MS, Muir H, Hall R. Perioperative management of drug therapy: clinical considerations. *Drugs* 1996; 51: 238–259

Ure DS, Gillies MA, James KS. Safe use of remifentanil in a patient treated with the monoamine oxidase inhibitor phenelzine. *Br J Anaesth* 2000; 84: 414–418

---

7 | Sickle cell disease

This autosomal dominant condition primarily affects African, Mediterranean, Indian, Caribbean and Middle Eastern descendants. It can affect up to 10% of these groups. The specific mutation (replacement of glutamate by valine in the sixth amino acid sequence on the β chain of haemoglobin) causes the haemoglobin (Hb) molecules to become 'sticky', polymerize and to form tactoids when the Hb is de-oxygenated (HbS). The tactoids are insoluble and result in a change in the conformation of the cell membrane so that the cell adopts the characteristic sickle shape.

The process is reversible but is time dependent and causes haemolysis. The cells aggregate and block capillaries.

Diagnosis is made by a 'sickledex' test and then confirmatory electrophoresis to identify homozygous or heterozygous patients. The heterozygous form (sickle trait) has a normal life expectancy, normal Hb levels, no clinical signs and requires profound arterial desaturation before sickling occurs. In the homozygous form (sickle disease) 85–90% of the Hb is sickle haemoglobin (HbS) and sickling will occur even at normal mixed venous oxygen levels. The haemoglobin may be around 6.5–10 g dl^{-1}. Precipitating factors are hypoxaemia, increased plasma viscosity (because of dehydration, hypothermia or stasis) or acidosis. Acute sickling occurs in venules and is reversible by rapid rehydration, for example, but once red cell wall damage occurs it becomes irreversible. These patients have a chronic haemolytic anaemia and they often present with the extreme pain caused by a sickling event. Precipitation may be by a wide variety of conditions, such as pregnancy, while viral infections, especially parvovirus, may precipitate an anaplastic crisis. Infarction of organs occurs and can lead to strokes, massive lung damage, renal damage, aseptic necrosis of the femoral head and splenomegaly. The lungs are particularly vulnerable. Transfusion of normal Hb can provide some protection, especially if the HbS is about 40% of the total Hb.

Where the use of a tourniquet is absolutely necessary, it should be placed as peripherally as possible in a thoroughly exsanguinated limb and for the shortest interval.

The postoperative period where oxygenation may be impaired is a particularly dangerous time and these patients should have supplementary oxygen. Abdominal or other major surgery mandates good analgesia and protection from hypoventilation and hypoxia.

Further reading

Esseltine DG, Baxter MR, Bevan JC. Sickle cell states and the anaesthetist. *Can J Anaesth* 1988; 35: 385–403

Frietsch T, Ewen I, Waschke KF. Anaesthetic care for sickle cell disease. *Eur J Anaesthesiol* 2001; 18: 137–150

Lanigan C, Justins D. Sickle cell crisis and pain management. *Anaesthesia* 1993; 48: 829–830

---

8   The anaesthetic implications of severe obesity

Severe obesity is defined as a body mass index (BMI = kg m^{-2}) greater than 30 and worldwide affects 30% of the population. Morbid obesity is a BMI > 35 and affects only about 1% of the population. Relevant physiological changes relate to the cardiovascular system, where there is increased blood volume, left ventricular hypertrophy, hypertension, increased oxygen consumption and cardiac autonomic dysfunction leading to a risk of sudden death. Respiratory changes include airway problems from the increased bulk of the soft tissues. There is increased work in breathing, ventilation–perfusion mismatching leading to large shunt values, and a high incidence of obstructive sleep apnoea; also the reduced functional residual capacity and the increased oxygen consumption lead to rapid and profound arterial desaturation. There are changes in the gut, with a very high resting level of gastric fluid and a low pH. There is frequently an impaired lower oesophageal sphincter tone and a hiatus hernia. Glucose intolerance, hyperlipidaemia and occult malignancies compound the picture.

Acid aspiration prophylaxis is advisable. Anaesthetic management includes securing the airway, good i.v. access and controlled ventilation if a general anaesthetic is chosen. Regional techniques are ideal but are often technically challenging. Sedative or opiate premedication can be fatal and an awake endotracheal intubation is usually advocated. Arterial gas monitoring should be used to supplement the routine invasive perioperative monitoring. Drug administration is best calculated from the 'ideal' BMI, not the actual, and lipophilic anaesthetic drugs are best avoided. Desflurane would appear to be the ideal volatile agents, but there is only limited data available at present. Admission to a high-dependency unit or critical care area is essential following surgery, as it will take time for complete recovery from the effects of the anaesthetic drugs. Prolonged ventilatory support will be necessary and use of a near-sitting position will be helpful. Analgesia with local anaesthetics offers optimal recovery without the risk of respiratory depression from opiate infusions. Infection and deep venous thrombosis are much more common complications and prophylactic antibiotics and heparin are advisable.

Further reading

Hunter JD, Reid C, Noble D. Anaesthetic management of the morbidly obese patient. *Hosp Med* 1998; 59: 481–483

Oberg B, Poulsen TD. Obesity: an anaesthetic challenge. *Acta Anaesthesiol Scand* 1996; 40: 191–200

9 Anaesthesia in a patient with myasthenia gravis

Myasthenia gravis is an autoimmune-mediated disease causing muscle weakness of both skeletal and bulbar muscles. It is due to the production of antibodies to the post-junctional acetylcholine receptors. There is progressive loss of power on exercise and it is believed that this is due to autoimmune damage to the neuromuscular junction. There may be both respiratory and bulbar weakness. Preoperative assessment must include respiratory function testing, confirmation of adequate cough, gas and swallowing reflexes. The associated conditions of thyroid disease, rheumatoid arthritis, systemic lupus erythematosus and polymyositis must be sought. Drug therapy often includes steroids, in high doses, and pyridostigmine. All these drugs must be continued throughout the perioperative period.

Plasmapheresis may be used to prepare the patient. Regional techniques should be used where possible. Perioperative management requires a protected airway because of the increased gastric volumes and acidity from the anticholinesterase therapy. Depolarizing agents, such as suxamethonium, should be avoided wherever possible and non-depolarizing agents used with extreme care. Titration of onset of block using cisatracurium or mivacurium may allow a minimal dose to be used.

Alternatively the use of volatile agents may be used to avoid muscle relaxants. Prior to extubation the efficiency of ventilation must be assessed and supported if necessary. There appears to be no 'ideal' anaesthetic agent and all volatile and intravenous agents are suitable. Regional techniques can prove hazardous if the height of the block extends into levels that include intercostal innervations. Postoperative care is very important, with particular attention to respiratory function.

Further reading

Baraka A. Anaesthesia and myasthenia gravis. *Can J Anaesth* 1992; 39: 476–486

Gambling DR. Anaesthesia and myasthenia gravis. *Can J Anaesth* 1992; 39: 1002–1003

10   Post-herpetic neuralgia

Post-herpetic neuralgia is one of the most common types of neurogenic pain seen in the pain clinic. About 50% of older patients with herpes zoster will develop post-herpetic neuralgia and this most commonly affects the trigeminal nerve, then the thoracic and lumbar segments and less commonly the limbs. Treatment of the acute phase with, for example, acyclovir, analgesia or sympathectomy may influence subsequent symptoms. The chronic pain has three characteristic components: a constant deep ache, sharp lancinating pain and severe dysaesthesia provoked by light tactile stimulation. The patient may then be in one of three broad groups: pain of short duration, chronic pain lasting a couple of years but decreasing, or continuous and unremitting pain.

The mainstay of treatment is amitriptyline, but carbamazepine and other anti-epileptic drugs may help lancinating pains. All types of nerve blocks have been tried with and without steroids, but there is no evidence that central blockade is more beneficial. Opioids may help the deep ache, but in general the side effects outweigh the benefits. Many stimulation techniques are used, including transcutaneous electrical nerve stimulation (TENS), acupuncture, vibration, ultrasound and capsaicin cream.

Further reading

Rowbotham MC. Managing post-herpetic neuralgia with opioids and local anesthetics. *Ann Neurol* 1994; 35(Suppl): S46–S49

11   Pudendal nerve block

Bilateral pudendal nerve blockade abolishes sensation in most of the perineum, vulva and vagina. The uterus is not anaesthetized. The main indication for its use is during the second stage of labour. It is usually administered by the obstetrician. Once venous access is established there are two methods. The transperineal method involves the insertion of a 100 mm, 22-gauge needle approximately halfway between the ischial tuberosity and the margin of the anal sphincter, directing the needle through the ischiorectal fossa to just behind the ischial spine and, following aspiration, injection of 10 ml of local anaesthetic. The more successful method is transvaginal, with the needle guided posteriorly by the fingers and placed just beyond the ischial spine. Effective block is shown by failure of the external anal sphincter to contract when touched. Complications include local anaesthetic toxicity from dose used or from intravascular placement, infection, laceration and failure (50%).

Further reading

Tetzschner T, Sorensen M, Rasmussen OO, Lose G, Christiansen J. Pudendal nerve damage increases the risk of fecal incontinence in women with anal sphincter rupture after childbirth. *Acta Obstet Gynecol Scand* 1995; 74: 434–440

12 pHi (gastric tonometry)

The gastric tonometer allows the measurement of gastric intramucosal pH. Practically, the tonometer is a gas-impermeable tube, at the end of which is a gas-permeable balloon that can be filled with saline. The tonometer is sited in the stomach, saline is introduced into the balloon and a period of time is allowed for the CO_2 in the tissues of the mucosa to equilibrate with the saline in the balloon. The saline is then aspirated anaerobically and the partial pressure of the CO_2 it contains assessed in a blood gas analyser. This value can be substituted into a modified version of the Henderson–Hasselbalch equation along with a bicarbonate level from a simultaneously taken arterial blood gas. The intramucosal pH (or pHi) can then be calculated. A low value (such as less than 7.32) indicates that perfusion is inadequate and that one should take measures to ensure an increased perfusion.

The concept of the tonometer facilitates the assessment of perfusion in the stomach, which in turn should provide an indication of the regional circulation of the gut.

It has been postulated that the loss of the integrity of the gut wall and the subsequent entry into the circulation of organisms and endotoxin is thought to precipitate the systemic inflammatory response syndrome (SIRS), which may progress to organ dysfunction and death. Ischaemic injury to the gut wall is thought to be the precipitating factor in the loss of its integrity. This technique allows this to be identified and measured.

There are, however, several problems with this technique. CO_2 is formed within the stomach when it releases acid, or bicarbonate refluxes from the duodenum. This falsely elevates the partial pressure of CO_2 in the balloon, causing the calculated pHi to be falsely low. The administration of the H_2-blocker ranitidine increases the accuracy of the tonometer by preventing acid secretion. Further, the assumption that the arterial and mucosal bicarbonate levels are the same is not necessarily correct. In circumstances such as occlusion to the arterial supply of the gut, the mucosal bicarbonate will be lower than that of the general circulation, making the calculation inaccurate. From a practical viewpoint the method is slow as equilibration has to take place, and it is also labour intensive. Despite these problems, in many circumstances tonometry is a relatively non-invasive method of assessing perfusion of the gut and can help in the intensive care management of patients.

There are now automated tonometers which allow more rapid equilibration and automated measurement, making the device far easier to use.

Further reading

Hamilton MA, Mythen MG. Gastric tonometry: where do we stand? *Curr Opin Crit Care* 2001; 7: 122–127

Mas A, Saura P, Joseph D, Blanch L, Baigorri F, Artigas A, Fernandez R. Effect of acute moderate changes in $PaCO_2$ on global hemodynamics and gastric perfusion. *Crit Care Med* 2000; 28: 360–365

Write short notes on the following topics. Do not miss out any questions and remember that there are only 3 hours in total to complete this paper.

1 Deep venous thrombosis prophylaxis

2 Tramadol

3 Anaesthesia for a minor gynaecological procedure in a lung transplant recipient

4 List the advantages of regional anaesthesia over general anaesthesia for eye surgery. State the contraindications for regional anaesthesia

5 Outline the mechanisms of phantom limb pain post amputation

6 The potential complications specific to 'needle through needle' combined spinal epidural anaesthesia

7 How would you perform a percutaneous tracheostomy on a ventilated ICU patient?

8 How would you gain consent for epidural analgesia for labour?

9 Heparin-induced thrombocytopenia

10 Discuss morbidity and mortality associated with regional and general anaesthesia for hip fracture surgery in the elderly patient

11 Write short notes on the therapeutic applications of magnesium

12 The causes and symptoms of peripheral neuropathies

Deep venous thrombosis (DVT) is difficult to diagnose clinically and essentially the only effective treatment is prevention. Pulmonary embolism accounts for the deaths of two in every 1000 postoperative patients but also has a very high incidence in medical patients. The risk factors for DVT can essentially be divided into background factors, disease or surgical factors. Increasing age, immobility, obesity, varicose veins, pregnancy or oestrogen treatments, or a past history of thromboembolism or various haematological disorders, e.g. antithrombin III deficiency, or phospholipid antibody syndrome, both of which constitute an increased risk, as does trauma, malignancy (especially pelvic or below), heart failure, recent myocardial infarction, paralysis and sepsis. Identifying which of these factors are relevant enables stratification into low-, medium-, and high-risk groups and appropriately directed therapy. Low-risk patients should not be exposed to the hazards and costs of antithrombotic drugs, but will benefit from compression stockings and early mobilization. At the other end of the scale, trials have shown the benefits in hip surgery of a variety of therapies including compression stockings, pneumatic devices, unfractionated heparins, low-molecular-weight heparins, adjusted-dose warfarin and intravenous dextran. The timing of initiating low-molecular-weight heparin has an influence on effectiveness. Therefore it should be given early. When anticoagulants are contraindicated, for example, in cerebral or spinal trauma, pneumatic devices should be used until the patient is ambulant.

Further reading

Breddin HK. Prophylaxis and treatment of deep-vein thrombosis. *Semin Thromb Hemost* 2000; 26: 47–52

Hull RD, Pineo GF, Stein PD, Mah AF et al. Timing of initial administration of low-molecular-weight heparin prophylaxis against deep vein thrombosis in patients following elective hip arthroplasty: a systematic review. *Arch Intern Med* 2001; 161: 1952–1960

Tramadol hydrochloride is a synthetic, centrally acting analgesic agent. It has two synergistic mechanisms of action. It is a weak opioid agonist but it also inhibits monoamine neurotransmitter reuptake.

Tramadol is rapidly absorbed after oral administration, with a bioavailability of 70%. Peak plasma levels are reached after 2 hours (5 hours with sustained-release capsules). Analgesia onset and peak plasma levels are similar after intramuscular administration. The majority is metabolized in the liver. There are five major metabolites, only one of which has analgesic activity. It has been shown to effectively relieve moderate to severe postoperative pain associated with surgery. Analgesic efficacy is similar to morphine or alfentanil.

Tramadol is an effective analgesia in both children and adults for inpatient and day surgery. It is well tolerated but the most common adverse events are nausea, dizziness, drowsiness, sweating, vomiting and dry mouth. Unlike other opioids it has very few clinically relevant effects on respiratory or cardiovascular parameters and a low potential for abuse or dependence. Most importantly, unlike other opioids, tramadol has no clinically relevant effects on respiratory or cardiovascular parameters. It is useful in patients with poor cardiopulmonary function, including the elderly, the obese and smokers, and in patients with impaired hepatic or renal function.

Further reading

Duthie DJ. Remifentanil and tramadol. *Br J Anaesth* 1998; 81: 51–57

Shipton EA. Tramadol – present and future. *Anaesth Intensive Care* 2000; 28: 363–374

---

3 | **Anaesthesia for a minor gynaecological procedure in a lung transplant recipient**

The problems are those relating to a combination of potentially impaired lung function and immunosuppression.

Pulmonary function. The patient may have one or two transplanted lungs. If they have had a double transplant then lung function is likely to be close to normal. Particularly in the early months post transplant there is likely to be some restrictive spirometric changes. Graft denervation results in impaired cough reflex (absent if a double transplant) and a reduction in mucociliary clearance.

Haematological system. Anaemia is common due to immunosuppression, iron deficiency or occult bleeding.

Nervous system. Complications include autonomic neuropathy.

Immunosuppression. Increases risk of infective complications. Drugs have many side effects, including:

- Impaired renal function.
- Blood dyscrasias.
- Interactions with other drugs.

Investigations should include:

- ECG.
- Chest X-ray.
- Spirometry.
- Full blood count.

- Electrolytes.
- Cyclosporin/tacrolimus levels.

Premedication

- Anxiolysis if required.
- Continue all immunosuppressants.
- Consider steroid therapy.
- Consider antibiotic prophylaxis.

Monitoring

Full standard monitoring; avoid invasive monitoring where possible to minimize infective risk.

Airway

- Proliferation of lymphoid tissue may result in airway obstruction.
- Tracheal stenosis or tracheomalacia may be present around sutures. If a tracheal tube is used it should not be advanced too far to avoid disrupting suture lines.
- Excessive airway pressures should be avoided for the same reason.

Anaesthetic technique

General anaesthesia. All standard intravenous induction and inhalational agents can be used safely. For short gynaecological procedures a spontaneously breathing technique is satisfactory. If muscle relaxants are used, neuromuscular function should be monitored as immunosuppressants may interfere with the pharmacokinetics of these drugs.

Regional anaesthesia. Assuming no bleeding tendency is present, a regional technique would be a suitable alternative. Cautious fluid loading should be used to minimize the risk of pulmonary oedema, as lymphatic drainage is reduced.

Postoperative management

- Observe in a high-dependency unit.
- Chest physiotherapy may be beneficial. Early mobilization will help to prevent pulmonary complications.
- Analgesia can be provided with paracetamol and/or short-acting opioids.
- Avoid non-steroidal drugs because of their potential nephrotoxicity.

Further reading

Haddow GR. Anaesthesia for patients after lung transplantation. *Can J Anaesth* 1997; 44: 182–197

4	List the advantages of regional anaesthesia over general anaesthesia for eye surgery. State the contraindications for regional anaesthesia

Regional anaesthesia advantages

- Minimal equipment required.
- Faster recovery.
- Superior postoperative pain control.
- Blockade of oculocardiac reflex.
- Avoid consequences of general anaesthesia.
- Less physiological trespass.
- Less postoperative nausea and vomiting.
- Full mental status retained.
- No risk of malignant hyperpyrexia.
- No risk of toxic hepatitis.
- No pollution.

Regional anaesthesia contraindications

- Informed patient refusal.
- Uncorrected, reversible medical condition.
- Anaesthetist inexperience.
- Surgeon preference for general anaesthesia.
- Prolonged surgery.
- Emergency surgery.
- Difficulty cooperating.
- Children.
- Unsuitable psychological status.
- Dementia.
- Inability to lie flat.
- Head movements/tremor.
- Intractable cough.
- Communication barrier.
- Needle phobia.
- Previous regional block complication.
- Patients with high myopia.
- Caution with patients on anticoagulants.

Further reading

Hamilton RC. Techniques of orbital regional anaesthesia. *Br J Anaesth* 1995; 75(1): 88–92

Seppelt I. Local anaesthesia for eye surgery. *Anaesth Intensive Care*. 1995; 23(4): 516

5 Outline the mechanisms of phantom limb pain post amputation

Phantom pain occurs in about 60–80% of patients following limb amputation but is only severe in about 5–10% of cases. The mechanisms involve factors in both the peripheral and central nervous system.

Peripheral nerve injury leads to responses in the periphery, spinal cord and supraspinal levels that initiate and maintain phantom limb pain.

Periphery. Injured afferent nerves induce synthesis of neurotransmitters not previously produced by the cell and downregulate normal output. Spontaneous ectopic neuronal discharge occurs.

Spinal cord. Central sensitization amplifies neuronal response to afferent input. The NMDA receptor is thought to be instrumental in its development.

Alterations in:

- Neurotransmitter production similar to periphery.
- Neurotransmitter receptor population within the spinal cord.
- Neuronal connections – sprouting of Aβ fibres into the dorsal horn induces pain on touch. Sympathetic fibre sprouting is also evident.

Supraspinal. Decrease in the inhibitory descending pathway activity, changes in somatosensory processing within the cortex. Accompanying emotional, affective and behavioural sequelae.

Further reading

Nikolajsen L, Staehelin-Jensen T. Phantom limb pain. *Curr Rev Pain* 2000; 4(2): 166–170

6 The potential complications specific to 'needle through needle' combined spinal epidural anaesthesia

Inadequate block

(a) Failure of spinal component

- Occurs in 2–5% of cases.
- Spinal needle may be too short to pass beyond the tip through the Tuohy needle or may be too long and pass through anterior dura.
- Long spinal needles mean delayed return of CSF, which may lead to incorrect diagnosis of failed dural puncture.
- If saline is used for epidural space identification, its return via spinal needle may be misinterpreted as CSF.
- The use of the Tuohy needle as an introducer results in a lack of 'feel' and dural puncture may occur unnoticed.

(b)   Failure of epidural component

This is no more common than with epidural as the sole component. However, inadequacies in the epidural block will not become apparent until the effects of spinal injection recede.

Subarachnoid placement of epidural catheter can occur:

- Via spinal needle hole at time of insertion.
- Via unrecognized dural puncture with Tuohy needle.
- If the catheter migrates though the dura after the inital placement.

This situation can be complicated by the fact that correct epidural catheter placement cannot be 'confirmed' by use of a test dose once subarachnoid drugs have been administered.

Nerve trauma

Potential for neural trauma as the epidural catheter is advanced, as warning paraesthesia is masked by spinal anaesthesia.

Delay in epidural catheter placement

There is inevitably some delay before completion of the procedure compared with spinal anaesthesia alone. The additional time required to insert and secure the epidural catheter can result in unintentionally high blocks if isobaric spinal solutions are used. If hyperbaric solutions are used then low or unilateral blocks may occur depending on patient position at time of insertion.

Further reading

Cook TM. Combined spinal–epidural techniques. *Anaesthesia* 2000; 55(1): 42–64

Rawal N et al. The combined spinal–epidural technique. *Anesthesiol Clin North Am* 2000; 18(2): 267–295

---

7   **How would you perform a percutaneous tracheostomy on a ventilated ICU patient?**

Explanation of procedure and consent – if patient condition allows. Usually discuss the necessity of the procedure with the family.

Equipment

- Choose the type of tracheostomy kit required and decide the size needed for tracheostomy but also drugs and equipment for conventional intubation.

Staff

- Operator plus suitably trained person responsible for sedation and airway control.

Fasting

- Routine preoperative fasting plus aspiration of oro/nasogastric tube prior to starting.

Anaesthesia

- Most agents suitable but i.v. induction/maintenance is useful in ICU setting. Neuromuscular relaxation. Full standard monitoring.

Ventilation

- 100% oxygen for at least 5 minutes prior to starting.
- Minute volume may need to be increased to compensate for leaks during the procedure.

Patient position

- Supine with sandbag under shoulders to maintain head extension.

Airway management

- Tracheal tube cuff deflated and tube withdrawn under direct vision until cuff is just distal to the cords.
- Alternatively, cuff can be withdrawn proximal to the cords and reinflated. A seal is maintained by gentle downward pressure of the cuff on the laryngeal inlet.

Skin preparation/incision

- Full aseptic technique.
- Local anaesthetic infiltration in midline at point midway between sternal notch and cricoid cartilage.
- Transverse skin incision just large enough for intended tracheostomy at above point.
- Blunt dissection of subcutaneous tissue down to trachea.

Tracheal location

- Insertion of needle or i.v cannula into tracheal lumen, in midline between 1st and 2nd or 2nd and 3rd tracheal rings.
- Placement confirmed by aspiration of air into saline filled syringe.

Flexible tipped guide wire passed via needle/cannula into trachea. Then run the short relatively stiff dilator down the wire and just into the trachea. Be careful not to push it in too far.

Three techniques are available which are identical until this stage. Thereafter the procedure is as follows:

Ciaglia technique

- Size 8 French gauge (FG) guiding catheter introduced over the guidewire.
- Dilatation of stoma using sequential dilators up to 36 FG which are advanced through the tracheal wall with the guiding catheter and guidewire.
- Tracheostomy tube is loaded on to appropriate size dilator and is passed into trachea as above.
- Guidewire, guiding catheter and dilator are removed.
- Tracheostomy cuff is inflated, the tracheostomy is secured and the breathing system connected.

Griggs technique

- Modified Howard Kelly forceps are passed over the guidewire into the trachea, with their jaws closed.
- The jaws are opened, spreading the soft tissues between the tracheal rings.
- The forceps are removed and a tracheostomy tube loaded on an introducer is advanced over the guidewire into the trachea.
- The guidewire and introducer are removed and the tracheostomy is secured and connected as above.
- Regardless of the technique, placement is verified by clinical observation (bilateral chest expansion) and by a characteristic capnograph trace. All patients should have a postoperative chest X-ray.

Blue rhino

There is a single dilator that increases gradually in diameter. It follows the wire and allows dilation in a single move.

In all these situations the newer tracheostomy tubes are easily placed then over the wire.

Further reading

Bennett MW, Bodenham AR. Percutaneous tracheostomy. *Clin Intensive Care* 1993; 4(6): 270–275

Grover A et al. Open versus percutaneous dilatational tracheostomy: efficacy and cost analysis. *Am Surg* 2001; 67(4): 297–302

Heafield S, Rogers R, Karnik A. Tracheostomy management in ordinary wards. *Hosp Med* 1999; 60(4): 261–262

Reeve IR. Percutaneous tracheostomy. In: Kaufman L, Ginsburg R (eds). *Anaesthesia Review* 15. Churchill Livingstone, Edinburgh, 1999: 169–183

8 How would you gain consent for epidural analgesia for labour?

This question is asking for the criteria necessary for informed consent prior to epidural analgesia. Consent involves presentation of medical information (disclosure) in a manner that is understood (patient competency) and which enables the patient to make an informed choice (decision-making). Whether a labouring mother is in a position to carry out these processes is open to debate. Similarly, if the anaesthetist fails to ensure completion of the process, then informed consent may not have been achieved. Written and verbal consent are equally valid, although subsequent recall may be better if written consent is obtained.

Areas to be covered in the discussion should include the following:

- Alternative options for analgesia during labour.
- General anaesthesia may be required in certain circumstances.
- The process of siting an epidural catheter.
- The incidence of failure (approx. 5%).
- The risk of post-dural puncture headache (approx. 1%).
- The risk of nerve damage or paralysis is one in 10 000, and although most problems resolve within days some may be permanent.
- Other rare complications may occur and could be life threatening.

Further reading

Gerancher JC, Grice SC, Dewon DM, Eisenbach J. An evaluation of informed consent prior to epidural analgesia for labour and delivery. *Int J Obstet Anaesth* 2000; 9: 168–173

9 Heparin-induced thrombocytopenia

There are two recognized forms:

Type 1

- Non-immune origin.
- Clinically insignificant, requiring no therapy.
- Presents within 4 days of therapy.

Type 2

- Severe thrombocytopenia with paradoxical thrombosis.
- Usually after at least 5 days' therapy.
- Haemorrhage is rare.

Heparin-induced thrombocytopenia (HIT) is thought to be caused by IgG antibodies that recognize complexes of heparin and platelet factor 4. This leads to platelet activation via platelet Fcγ IIa receptors and the formation of platelet-derived microparticles which aggregate and cause thrombosis. Diagnosis can be made when one or more typical clinical events (most frequently, thrombocytopenia with or without thrombosis) occur in a patient with detectable HIT antibodies.

The incidence of HIT has been quoted as high as 1–5% of surgical patients and as many as 35% of these patients may experience HIT and thrombosis syndrome (HITTS). Clinically, these patients present with very low platelet counts and acute, sometimes severe, haemorrhage. Treatment is restricted to withdrawal of the drug and symptomatic treatment of bleeding.

Further reading

Kaplan KL, Francis CW. Heparin-induced thrombocytopenia. *Blood Rev* 1999; 13(1): 1–7

10	Discuss morbidity and mortality associated with regional and general anaesthesia for hip fracture surgery in the elderly patient

Hip fracture surgery is a common procedure with increasing incidence. The mean age for recipients requiring hip fracture repair is approximately 80 years. Patients in this population frequently present with significant coexisting disease. Morbidity and mortality are accordingly high with figures of a 12-month mortality of 26% being recorded. Men had a higher mortality rate than women for all fracture types that was independent of age.

Regardless of the method of anaesthesia to be used, expeditious surgery following comprehensive assessment and appropriate resuscitation on presentation are desirable clinical goals.

Controversy continues with regard to choice of anaesthesia for hip fracture surgery, indicating that differences in outcome are marginal. A recent meta-analysis (see below) has revealed advantages for regional anaesthesia compared to general anaesthesia in terms of 1-month mortality (6.4% vs. 9.4%) and risk of deep venous thrombosis (30.2% vs. 46.9%). A tendency towards a lower incidence for perioperative confusion (12.0% vs. 22.6%), hypoxia (35.7% vs. 48.3%) and myocardial infarction (0.9% vs. 1.8%) also favoured regional anaesthesia. However, the incidence of intraoperative hypotension was lower and the operative time was shorter in the general anaesthesia group. The method of airway maintenance and ventilation for general anaesthesia had no impact on outcome measures. Similarly, there was no difference between regional and general anaesthesia for the incidence of pneumonia, urinary retention, postoperative nausea and vomiting and blood transfusion requirements.

Further reading

O'Hara DA, Duff A, Berlin JA, Poses RM, Lawrence VA, Huber EC, Noveck H, Strom BL, Carson JL. The effect of anesthetic technique on postoperative outcomes in hip fracture repair. *Anesthesiology* 2000; 92(4): 947–957

Urwin SC, Parter MJ, Griffiths R. General versus regional anaesthesia for hip fracture surgery: a meta-analysis of randomized trials. *Br J Anaesth* 2000; 84: 450–455

11   Write short notes on the therapeutic applications of magnesium

Magnesium deficiency

- Serum levels do not accurately reflect magnesium stores, so diagnosis is difficult.

Pregnancy-induced hypertension

- Treatment and prevention of seizures in eclampsia/severe pre-eclampsia.
- To obtund the pressor response to laryngoscopy.

Cardiac arrhythmias; often used as empirical treatment

- Treatment of many ventricular and supraventricular arrhythmias.
- Prevention of arrhythmias after cardiopulmonary bypass.

Induced hypotension

- Blood pressure decreased by vasodilation.
- Cardiac output maintained without reflex tachycardia.

Myocardial infarction

- May limit infarct size and improve survival if given at time of acute event.

Tetanus

- Limits sympathetic overactivity.
- Gives degree of muscle relaxation.

Phaeochromocytoma

- Inhibits catecholamine release from adrenal medulla.
- Vasodilation and decreased blood pressure.

Severe asthma

- Bronchodilatory properties if given intravenously or by inhalation.

Further reading

Idama TO, Lindow SW. Magnesium sulphate: a review of clinical pharmacology applied to obstetrics. *Br J Obstet Gynaecol* 1998; 105(3): 260–268

Murphy N. Magnesium in anaesthesia and intensive care. In: *Anaesthesia Review 15*. Churchill Livingstone, Edinburgh, 1999: 47–61

Rowe BH, Bretzlaff JA, Bourdon C, Bota GW, Camargo CA. Intravenous magnesium sulfate treatment for acute asthma in the emergency department: a systematic review of the literature. *Ann Emerg Med* 2000; 36(3): 181–190

Shechter M, Hod H, Kaplinsky E, Rabinowitz B. The rationale of magnesium as alternative therapy for patients with acute myocardial infarction without thrombolytic therapy. *Am Heart J* 1996; 132(2 Pt 2 Suppl): 483–486, discussion 496–502

---

12   **The causes and symptoms of peripheral neuropathies**

Damage to nerves in the periphery induces increased afferent signals. This induces central wind-up. These damaged axons then become hypersensitive. The type of nerve fibre damaged has a bearing on the symptoms experienced. Bilateral symmetrical symptoms are usually the result of systemic causes.

Causes and symptoms

- Diabetic neuropathy. Small fibres principally affected with pain, burning and autonomic instability. Pain in diabetics may also be due to peripheral vascular disease, joint pain and ulcers.
- Alcoholic neuropathy. Can occur in the absence of vitamin deficiency. Damage is non-selective with sensory and motor deficit.
- Nutritional neuropathies. Niacin and B_1 deficiency can cause a painful neuropathy. Burning feet is not a neuropathy as such but responds to B vitamins.

Infections such as leprosy produce a polyneuritis multiplex that affects sensory motor and autonomic nerves.

Other causes

Isoniazid, statins, hypothyroidism, myeloma, AIDS and chronic renal failure. Some of the antiretrovirals also cause both myopathy and neuropathy; nucleoside analogue reverse transcriptase inhibitors (NRTIs).

Further reading

Perkins AT, Morgenlander JC. Endocrinologic causes of peripheral neuropathy: pins and needles in a stocking-and-glove pattern and other symptoms. *Postgrad Med* 1997; 102(3): 81–82, 90–92, 102–106

Paper Two Write short notes on the following topics. Do not miss out any questions and remember that there are only 3 hours in total to complete this paper.

1 List the advantages and disadvantages of general and regional anaesthetic techniques for carotid endarterectomy

2 List the possible complications from subclavian vein cannulation. Describe how to avoid them

3 Describe how critical illness neuropathy is distinguished from Guillain–Barré syndrome. How is critical illness neuropathy treated?

4 Write short notes on the anaesthetic management of a 28-year-old pregnant woman undergoing a craniotomy and clipping of an intracranial aneurysm

5 Anaesthesia for renal transplantation

6 What are the indications for renal replacement therapy in ICU? Outline the techniques used in this setting

7 What are the physiological changes that follow a rapid loss of 20% of blood volume in an adult?

8 Discuss the increased risk of anaesthesia in patients with Down's syndrome

9 Draw an algorithm for basic life support of the newborn

10 The action of suxamethonium at the neuromuscular junction

11 Methods of measuring the FiO_2 commonly available in theatre

12 What are the indications for and the contraindications to epidural blood patch? Outline how you would perform such a procedure

List the advantages and disadvantages of general and regional anaesthetic techniques for carotid endarterectomy

General anaesthesia: advantages

- Airway control throughout the procedure.
- Tight control of arterial PCO_2.
- Cerebral protection by barbiturates.
- Ability to induce hypothermia if required.

General anaesthesia: disadvantages

- Difficulty in monitoring cerebral perfusion during cross-clamping.
- Potential for cerebral blood 'steal' phenomenon with isoflurane.
- High concentration of volatile are required for cerebral protection.
- Cardiovascular instability is common.
- Postoperative nausea and vomiting.

Regional anaesthesia: advantages

- Patient's mental state is an excellent monitor of cerebral perfusion.
- Low requirement for internal carotid artery shunting.
- Lower cardiovascular morbidity.
- Shorter hospital stay and less overall expense.
- Avoidance of intubation in patients with pulmonary disease.
- Better autoregulation of cerebral circulation.

Regional anaesthesia: disadvantages

- Relatively complex techniques with their own complications.
- Potential for failed or patchy blocks.
- Local anaesthetic toxicity from excessive dosage or misplaced injection.
- Potential for conversion to general anaesthesia in a patient with a compromised cerebral circulation.
- Myocardial ischaemia is not prevented.
- High degree of patient cooperation required.

Further reading

Stoneharn MD, Knighton JD. Regional anaesthesia for carotid endarterectomy. *Br J Anaesth* 1999; 82: 910–919

 List the possible complications from subclavian vein cannulation. Describe how to avoid them

Complications

- Air embolism.
- Pneumothorax.

- Subclavian artery puncture.
- Haematoma.
- Haemothorax.
- Thoracic duct injury.
- Sepsis.

Avoidance of complications

Optimize the patient's positioning by placing a small towel or pillow between the patient's scapulae and ensure the ipsilateral arm is by the patient's side. Prevent air embolism by positioning the patient head down. Use a sterile technique and carefully prepare the skin to minimize risk of introducing infection.

Identify the landmarks

The point of entry should be 1 cm below the medial and middle third of the clavicle. Use the Seldinger technique and take care to avoid damaging other structures by guiding the tip of the needle under the clavicle in the direction of the suprasternal notch. Aspirate the catheter to test for intravascular placement. Attach the catheter to a pressure waveform monitor and ensure a central venous pressure trace is present. Finally order and examine a chest X-ray to confirm position of the catheter tip and to exclude presence of pneumo- or haemothorax. Be aware that a pneumothorax may take some hours to become clinically or radiologically apparent.

Further reading

Henriques HF III, Karmy-Jones R, Knoll SM, Copes WS, Giordano JM. Avoiding complications of long-term venous access. *Am Surg* 1993; 59(9): 555–558

Reed CR, Sessler CN, Glauser FL, Phelan BA. Central venous catheter infections: concepts and controversies. *Intensive Care Med* 1995; 21(2): 177–183

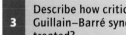

3 Describe how critical illness neuropathy is distinguished from Guillain–Barré syndrome. How is critical illness neuropathy treated?

- History and examination offer little to distinguish these two conditions. Both produce flaccid, areflexic paralysis precipitated by a period of illness.
- There are two tests that aid diagnosis. Firstly, neurophysiological studies can identify axonal loss caused by critical illness neuropathy. Stimulation of the nerves leads to a reduction in the amplitude of the transmitted signal rather than slowing of the signal, which is seen in Guillain–Barré, secondary to

demyelination. Secondly, examination of cerebrospinal fluid (CSF) reveals normal CSF in critical illness neuropathy. Guillain–Barré produces CSF with increased protein and no cells.
- Treatment is supportive. Prolonged weaning from assisted ventilation should be anticipated.

Further reading

Coakley JH, Nagendran K, Honavar M, Hinds CJ. Preliminary observations on the neuromuscular abnormalities in patients with organ failure and sepsis. *Intensive Care Med* 1993; 19: 323–328

Hund EF, Borel CO, Cornblath DR, Hanley DF, McKhann GM. Intensive management and treatment of severe Guillain–Barré syndrome. *Crit Care Med* 1993; 21(3): 433–446

---

4 **Write short notes on the anaesthetic management of a 28-year-old pregnant woman undergoing a craniotomy and clipping of an intracranial aneurysm**

The following points should be included:

Preoperative assessment

- Full history/examination.
- Particular attention to effects of pregnancy on subarachnoid haemorrhage.
- Obtain consent including explanation of risks of inducing preterm labour.

Premedication

- Anxiolysis if required.
- Aspiration prophylaxis.
- Discuss with obstetrician concerning prophylactic tocolysis.

Monitoring

- Routine monitoring for craniotomy plus cardiotocograph.

Intraoperative management

- Aim to maintain maternal and fetal tissue perfusion.
- In particular, avoid hypoxia, hypotension and hyperventilation.

Induction

- Rapid-sequence induction with cricoid pressure.
- Thiopentone/etomidate are safe but propofol can also probably be used.
- Small-diameter endotracheal tube, as respiratory tract mucosa may be engorged.

Maintenance

- All modern volatile agents are acceptable.
- Nitrous oxide is controversial but probably safe.
- High FiO_2 to avoid hypoxia.
- IPPV.
- Non-depolarizing muscle relaxants are safe.
- If deliberate hypotension is required monitor fetus.
- Avoid marked hyperventilation.

Postoperatively

- Routine maternal care.
- Continue monitoring fetus for 24 hours postoperatively.

Further reading

Hawkins JL. *Anesthesis for the Pregnant Patient Undergoing Non Obstetric Surgery. Refresher Courses in Anesthesiology*, Vol. 25. American Society of Anesthesiologists, 1997

Kriplani A, Relan S, Misra NK, Mehta VS, Takkar D. Ruptured intracranial aneurysm complicating pregnancy. *Int J Gynaecol Obstet* 1995; 48(2): 201–206

Stoodley MA, Macdonald RL, Weir BK. Pregnancy and intracranial aneurysms. *Neurosurg Clin North Am* 1998; 9(3): 549–556

5   Anaesthesia for renal transplantation

Preoperative assessment

The patient may well be on dialysis so details concerning the last dialysis, current fluid status and metabolic status are important and relevant.

Particular attention should be paid to coexisting disorders that may be the cause or effect of the renal failure. These include:

- Diabetes.
- Atheromatous diseases.
- Hypertension.
- Heart failure.
- Autoimmune diseases.

The patient is likely to be on multiple medications, and the potential effects of these should be taken into account.

Other important preoperative factors

- *Fluid balance* – time since last dialysis, weight compared to ideal, acid/base status, electrolytes, particularly serum potassium.
- *Anaemia* – chronic anaemia is almost inevitable. Hb is likely to be between 6 and 8 g dl^{-1}. Consideration should be given to preoperative transfusion if lower than this.
- *Gastric emptying* is delayed in chronic renal failure, so local fasting guidelines should be observed.

Management of anaesthesia

The procedure may take up to 4 hours.

- *Premedication is* optional, but in view of poor gastric emptying antacid prophylaxis may be given.
- *Monitoring.* Routine standard monitoring plus central venous pressure to allow accurate monitoring of fluid balance. A peripheral nerve stimulator is also recommended. Temperature monitoring is also useful as the procedure may be prolonged.
- *Intravenous access.* Avoid limbs with arteriovenous fistula.
- *Induction.* All the standard induction agents are suitable. Some authorities recommend using a rapid-sequence induction.
- *Muscle relaxants.*
- Suxamethonium can be used in the absence of hyperkalaemia if necessary. Avoid suxamethonium if serum potassium is greater than 5.5 mmol l^{-1}. Atracurium has the advantage of Hofmann degradation, but vecuronium and *cis*-atracurium have also been used. Avoid pancuronium (and gallamine). Pharmacokinetics of relaxants are altered in these patients, so monitoring with nerve stimulator useful.
- *Maintenance.* Usually with volatiles but TIVA is also suitable. Isoflurane or desflurane is preferable because they undergo minimal biotransformation. Isoflurane is the volatile of choice due to low fluoride production. Enflurane is contraindicated because of the potential risk of renal toxicity from free fluoride ions.
- *Analgesia.* Fentanyl pharmacokinetics are affected little, so is useful intraoperatively or as PCA postoperatively. Morphine is suitable postoperatively but glucuronide metabolites may accumulate, prolonging clinical effects.
- *Fluid therapy.* Maintain good hydration, CVP 10–15 mmHg. Mannitol and/or frusemide before revascularization may improve graft survival.
- Warming and pressure care are important.

Postoperative care

- Ensure reversal of relaxation.
- Close attention to maintenance of intravascular volume. Aggressive treatment of hypo/hypertension.

- Check serum electrolytes.
- Despite the accumulation of its metabolites, morphine and postoperative PCA are ideal.

Further reading

Kirvela M, Scheinin M, Lindgren L. Haemodynamic and catecholamine responses to induction of anaesthesia and tracheal intubation in diabetic and non-diabetic uraemic patients. *Br J Anaesth* 1995; 74(1): 60–65

Norio K, Makisalo H, Isoniemi H, Groop PH, Pere P, Lindgren L. Are diabetic patients in danger at renal transplantation? An invasive perioperative study. *Eur J Anaesthesiol* 2000; 17(12): 729–736

---

6 | **What are the indications for renal replacement therapy in ICU? Outline the techniques used in this setting**

Indications for renal replacement therapy are:

- Severe uraemia.
- Uncontrollable hyperkalaemia.
- Severe salt and water overload.
- Severe acidosis.
- To accommodate fluid load of total parenteral nutrition or blood transfusion.

Techniques of renal replacement therapy. All variants of haemodialysis rely on the following features:

- Intravascular access (venous and/or arterial). This has to be large-bore to allow high flow.
- Extracorporeal circuit involving some form of artificial kidney.
- Anticoagulation.

Venovenous techniques have largely superseded arteriovenous ones for use in the critically ill.

Filtration

Here the blood is passed through the artificial kidney and fluid is drawn off using a highly permeable membrane, Replacement fluid is given to maintain circulating volume. This is a very efficient way of removing fluid.

Dialysis

Blood is passed on one side of a membrane and dialysis fluid on the other side. Equilibration occurs, removing metabolites from the circulation. This is the most efficient way of removing metabolites.

Haemodiafiltration

Combines the two processes, giving the advantages of both.

Venovenous techniques include:

- *Slow continuous ultrafiltration* (SCUF). Ultrafiltration is the convective transfer of fluid out of the plasma compartment via pores in the membrane. SCUF is removal of ultrafiltrate at rates below 5 ml min^{-1}. Mainly used in treatment of volume overload.
- *Continuous venovenous haemofiltration* (CVVHF). Removal of ultrafiltrate at higher rates than above (500 ml h^{-1}) with administration of replacement electrolyte solution. The clearance achieved approximates to the rate of fluid exchange, i.e. 500 ml h^{-1} is a clearance of 8.3 ml min^{-1}.
- *Continuous venovenous haemodiafiltration* (CVVHD). Dialysis is the removal of solute and fluid by their passage across a semipermeable membrane. Solutes pass by diffusion into the dialysate depending on their concentration gradient, size of molecule, permeability of the membrane and dialysis duration. Fluid is removed by exerting a hydrostatic pressure across the membrane. Advantages are that clearance may be quite efficient and is partially determined by dialysate flow. At 2 l min^{-1} dialysate flow and 140 ml min^{-1} blood flow clearances are usually of the order of 25 ml min^{-1}. However, as it is 'dialysis' very little fluid is actually removed. Additional solute passes across the membrane with this fluid (convective transport) and this method can be manipulated to adjust fluid removal. There is therefore a dialysis and a filtration component.
- *Peritoneal dialysis*. Large volumes of dialysis fluid are instilled into the peritoneal cavity. The peritoneum acts as the semipermeable membrane. It is rarely used in ICU.

Further reading

Bellomo R, Mansfield D, Rumble S, Shapiro J, Parkin G, Boyce N. A comparison of conventional dialytic therapy and acute continuous hemodiafiltration in the management of acute renal failure in the critically ill. *Ren Fail* 1993; 15(5): 595–602

van Bommel EF, Leunissen KM, Weimar W. Continuous renal replacement therapy for critically ill patients: an update. *J Intensive Care Med* 1994; 9(6): 265–280

---

7 | **What are the physiological changes that follow a rapid loss of 20% of blood volume in an adult?**

1   A fall in blood volume causes reduced venous return.

2   The fall in right atrial pressure and volume reduces the right ventricular stroke volume.

3   Reduced filling of the left side of the heart leads to a fall in cardiac output. The pulse pressure and systolic pressure fall.

4 A fall in systolic pressure leads to baroreceptor-initiated tachycardia, peripheral vasoconstriction, adrenaline secretion and redistribution of blood volume to the vital organs.

5 Antidiuretic hormone and aldosterone secretion leads to thirst, water retention, oliguria and water transfer from the extracellular fluid to the circulation.

6 Renin and angiotensin activity leads to further vasoconstriction.

7 Steroids are secreted as part of the stress response.

8 There is also increased movement of interstitial fluid to the intravascular compartment.

---

8   **Discuss the increased risk of anaesthesia in patients with Down's syndrome**

Down's syndrome is a common congenital abnormality associated with disorders of many organ systems with a broad spectrum of severity.

- A degree of mental retardation is present.
- There is an increased incidence postoperative agitation.
- Resistance to sedatives may complicate management.
- Muscle hypotonia reduces the ability to maintain an adequate airway. A degree of airway obstruction and sleep apnoea is common.
- Excess salivation, a large tongue and adenotonsillar hypertrophy are often present.
- Postoperative respiratory infections are frequent and associated with relative immune deficiency.
- Postoperative respiratory stridor occurs in a third of Down's syndrome patients.
- Congenital cardiac abnormalities can be significant; the majority involve a left-to-right shunt predisposing the child to pulmonary hypertension. Perioperative antibiotics may be required to prevent endocarditis.
- Increased sensitivity to atropine has been reported.
- Gastrointestinal abnormalities are a frequent reason for surgery early in life. Gastro-oesophageal reflux is found more often in this group.
- Atlanto-axial instability predisposes to subluxation and the risk of spinal cord compression.

Further reading

Mitchell V, Howard R, Facer E. Down's syndrome and anaesthesia. *Paediatr Anaesth* 1995; 5(6): 379–384

Morton RE, Khana MA, Murray-Leslie C, Elliott S. Atlantoaxial instability in Down's syndrome: a five year follow up study. *Arch Dis Child* 1995; 72(2): 115–119

9 Draw an algorithm for basic life support of the newborn

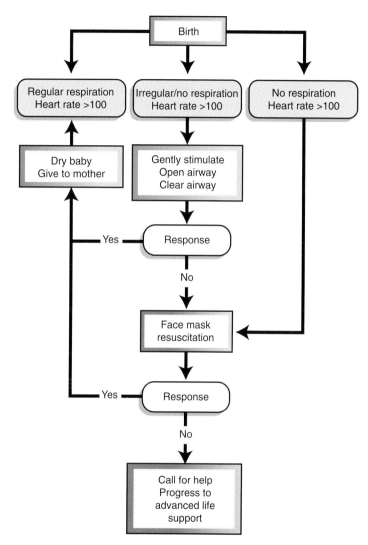

(After Ziderman, with permission from Oxford University Press.)

10   The action of suxamethonium at the neuromuscular junction

Suxamethonium is a depolarizing muscle relaxant that has a biphasic action on skeletal muscle. Initial depolarization and contraction (seen as fasciculation) are followed by relaxation. Initial depolarization is achieved by the interaction of the molecule with the acetylcholine receptor (AChR). This results in a wave of depolarization of the surrounding cell membrane and muscular contraction.

Why doesn't the continued presence of the suxamethonium in the synaptic cleft cause continued tetanic contraction of the muscle? Sodium channels have two gates (named voltage- and time-dependent), both of which need to be open for ion flux to occur. In the resting state, the voltage-dependent channel is closed and the time-dependent channel open. Depolarization causes the voltage-dependent channel to open and ion flux to occur. This is followed by closure of the time-dependent channel, regardless of voltage. Resetting of the channel to its resting stage requires restoration of voltage (and subsequent closure of the voltage-dependent gate) and then the time-dependent gate opens. The time-dependent gate remains closed until the voltage gate closes.

Following administration of suxamethonium, the AChR remains depolarized and so the voltage remains low in the surrounding sodium channels. This prevents resetting of the channels and results in an area of unresponsive sodium channels around the receptor. This prevents further contraction. Contraction can only occur once the suxamethonium has diffused away from the synaptic cleft.

11   Methods of measuring the FiO_2 commonly available in theatre

The main methods for measuring FiO_2 in anaesthetic gases are the fuel cell and paramagnetic analysis.

Fuel cell

This relies on the combination of oxygen with water and electrons to form hydroxyl ions at the gold cathode of the cell. Electrons are generated at a lead anode by the reaction lead with the hydroxyl ions. The current generated is proportional to the oxygen tension. This method has the advantage of being cheap but is affected by temperature and requires regular calibration.

Paramagnetic analysis

As a result of its atomic structure, oxygen, in contrast to most gases, is attracted towards a magnetic field (paramagnetic). Nitrogen is weakly diamagnetic. Oxygen measurement by paramagnetic means relies on a dumb-bell-shaped container of nitrogen being suspended in a chamber of test gas across which a magnetic field is applied. The higher the concentration of oxygen within the chamber, the greater the relative diamagnetic effect is on the nitrogen-filled dumb-bell. The dumb-bell is attached to a filament and rotation around this axis is measured using a light and mirror arrangement.

12 What are the indications for and the contraindications to epidural blood patch? Outline how you would perform such a procedure

Indications

- Treatment of moderate to severe post-dural puncture headache (PDPH).
- Prophylaxis of PDPH after unintentional dural puncture (controversial).
- Treatment of spontaneous low CSF pressure headache (Schaltenbrand's syndrome).

Contraindications

(a) Contraindications to needle placement:

- Patient refusal.
- Coagulopathy.
- Local or systemic sepsis.
- Anatomical distortion preventing epidural space identification.

(b) Contraindications to injection of blood:

- Systemic sepsis, proven or suspected (e.g. pyrexia).

Performance of epidural blood patch (EBP)

- *Timing.* Usually at least 24 hours after dural puncture, once headache is established and a trial of conservative management has failed. May be performed earlier if symptoms of PDPH are present and severe.
- *Explanation and consent.* A full explanation of the procedure, its risk (including repeat dural puncture) and benefits should be given and consent obtained.
- *Personnel.* Two operators plus an assistant are required.
- *Patient position.* Can be sitting but as headache is posture related the lateral position is preferred.
- *Epidural space localization.* Under strict aseptic conditions.
- *Venepuncture.* After epidural space is identified the second operator withdraws 20 ml of the patient's blood, again under strict aseptic conditions.
- *Injection of blood.* Slowly via Tuohy needle. Stop briefly after each 5 ml. Enquire about symptoms of back/leg pressure or pain. Stop injecting if symptoms develop. Injection can recommence if symptoms subside completely. Up to 20 ml can be injected but injecting more than 10 ml confers little benefit.
- *After-care.* The patient should remain supine for 2 hours after the procedure. It symptom free they can then be discharged.
- *Follow-up.* Instruct the patient to return if the headache returns or if visual or hearing difficulties develop.

Further reading

Choi A, Laurito CE, Cunningham FE. Pharmacologic management of postdural puncture headache. *Ann Pharmacother* 1996; 30(7–8): 831–839

Duffy PJ, Crosby ET. The epidural blood patch: resolving the controversies. *Can J Anesth* 1999; 46: 878–886

Ziderman DA. Resuscitation. *Br J Anaesth* 1999; 83(1): 157–168

Paper One Write short notes on the following topics. Do not miss out any questions and remember that there are only 3 hours in total to complete this paper.

1. Ventilator strategies in adult respiratory distress syndrome
2. Anaesthesia for removal of phaeochromocytoma
3. Drug–receptor interactions
4. Measures that can be taken to minimize central venous catheter-related infections
5. What physiological processes involve α_2-adrenergic receptors? Outline the investigated and potential clinical uses for α_2-agonists
6. List the potential neurological complications arising from obstetric regional anaesthesia
7. The physiological roles of albumin
8. The risks of anaesthetizing a premature infant
9. The common causes and effects of hypomagnesaemia
10. Zopiclone
11. The factors that influence the passive diffusion across cell membranes
12. The perioperative care of patients' eyes

1 Ventilator strategies in adult respiratory distress syndrome

Adult respiratory distress syndrome (ARDS) has had many definitions over the years. A practical way of looking at the problem is as an index of gas exchange. A commonly used criterion is a PaO_2/FiO_2 ratio of less than 200 mmHg (25 kPa).

Pathophysiology

Gattinoni described three zones in ARDS lung: normally aerated lung, potentially recruitable but partially collapsed and consolidated lung, and fully consolidated lung. Ventilator strategies aim to preserve normally aerated lung and recruit all potentially recruitable lung.

Strategies include the following:

- *PEEP*. this prevents closure of lung units, and their de-recruitment. Ideally it should be aimed at the inflection point on the compliance curve.
- *Small-volume ventilation*. This prevents barotrauma (which should more properly be called volutrauma).
- *Inverse ratio ventilation*. Allows recruitment of alveoli with differing time constants; provides further recruitment.
- *Permissive hypoxaemia and hypercapnia*. Involves allowing the PCO_2 to drift up in the absence of severe acidaemia and the PO_2 to be below 10 kPa when there is no evidence of poor oxygen delivery. This reduces the pressures and volumes needed to ventilate the patient.
- *Prone ventilation*. Works by a number of methods; the most obvious being a change in V/Q matching. The alveolar exudates on chest X-ray look homogeneous. On CT the exudate and consolidation occur in the posterior chest in the supine patient. By turning the patient prone, the exudates are transferred to the non-dependent position. This improves V/Q matching as the distribution of blood flow is determined by gravity, and also the weight of the lung recruits some of the consolidated lung, which explains the continued improvement after returning the patient to the supine position.

Further reading

Eisner MD, Thompson T, Hudson LD, Luce JM, Hayden D, Schoenfeld D, Matthay MA. Efficacy of low tidal volume ventilation in patients with different clinical risk factors for acute lung injury and the acute respiratory distress syndrome. *Am J Respir Crit Care Med* 2001; 164(2): 231–236

Meade MO, Cook DJ. The aetiology, consequences and prevention of barotrauma: a critical review of the literature. *Clin Intensive Care* 1995; 6(4): 166–173

Pinsky MR. Toward a better ventilation strategy for patients with acute lung injury. *Crit Care* 2000; 4(4): 205–206

2 Anaesthesia for removal of phaeochromocytoma

Phaeochromocytoma is a tumour of chromaffin tissue. The tumour may be benign or malignant, solitary or multiple, and may occur at any postganglionic site. It is occasionally associated with multiple endocrine neoplasia. The predominant problem is the presence of catecholamines: in variable amounts either adrenaline or noradrenaline.

Preoperative blockade should be started days before surgery. Suggested aims are that the blood pressure is < 160/90 for 24 hours prior to surgery, and that orthostatic hypotension is present with blood pressure of > 80/45. The ECG should be free of ST changes and no more than one VE/5 minutes should be present before surgery is commenced. Many anaesthetists prefer slow blockade with a non-competitive α-blocker, phenoxybenzamine, over 1–2 weeks that allows some readjustment of the intravascular volume. β-Blockade may be added in if required.

Conduct of anaesthesia

Invasive cardiovascular monitoring and large-bore intravenous access are mandatory. Histamine release should be avoided, but many different anaesthetic techniques to avoid stimulation and provide good operating conditions have been suggested.

Epidural anaesthesia

This has been shown to suppress the release of catecholamines during tumour manipulation.

Perioperative problems

Hypertension induced during tumour manipulation, where both glycerol trinitrate (GTN) and sodium nitroprusside have their advocates. Hypotension following tumour removal may require inotropic support occasionally.

Phentolamine, prazocin, labetalol, magnesium sulphate and esmolol have all been used to correct intraoperative hypertension. Hypotension seen postoperatively may respond to fluid but vasoconstrictors may be required.

Postoperatively

Postoperative care should be in a high-dependency environment. Postoperative drowsiness is common, possibly because of the removal of central catecholamine stimulation. Patients are sensitive to the effects of opioids. Postoperative epidural analgesia provides the most satisfactory analgesia.

Further reading

Prys-Roberts C. Phaeochromocytoma: recent progress in its management. *Br J Anaesth* 2000; 85(1): 44–57

Russell WJ, Metcalfe IR, Tonkin AL, Frewin DB. The preoperative management of phaeochromocytoma. *Anaesth Intensive Care* 1998; 26(2): 196–200

3 Drug–receptor interactions

Most receptors, with the exception of those for steroids, occur on cell surfaces. Binding of the drug to the receptor causes a conformational change in the receptor, which produces the biological change. Receptors exert their actions through three principal means:

1   *Changes in ionic permeability.* Receptor and ion channel are usually part of the same complex. Receptor occupancy causes a conformational change in the complex which results in a change in permeability, either to specific ions, e.g. the GABA receptor and Cl^- ions, or non-specifically, e.g. the acetylcholine receptor.

2   *Second messenger systems.* These allow amplification of the message. Receptor occupancy activates intracellular enzymes, which produce or reduce the amount of secondary messenger. The effect of the messenger is to phosphorylate proteins, which causes a change in their function and leads to the action of the drug. This can be due to changes in cell permeability (e.g. calcium in smooth muscle), ion channel effects or changes in DNA synthesis. There are four main second messenger systems in the body:

   • cAMP: activation of a G protein causes activation or inhibition of adenyl cyclase. This increases or decreases the amount of cAMP in the cell. Phosphodiesterase is responsible for the breakdown of cAMP. Phosphodiesterase inhibitors therefore act here.
   • cGMP: similar in action to cAMP.
   • Nitric oxide: produced by the vascular endothelium in response to shear stress, and by GTN, it interacts with guanyl cyclase, which converts GTP to cGMP. This leads to protein phosphorylation and reduced calcium entry, leading to vascular relaxation.
   • Phosphoinositides: interaction of drug with a different G protein causes activation of phospholipase C. This releases P1, P3 and diacyl glycerol. P1P3 causes increased calcium mobilization and either muscle contraction or the activation of calmodulin by a conformational change leading to changes in other enzymes. Diacyl glycerol activates protein kinases and therefore causes protein phosphorylation and activation.

3   *Changes in nucleic acid production.* Steroids are lipid soluble and diffuse into cells. The steroid then alters protein production by its interaction with DNA. Glucocortcoids cause an increase in lipocortin production. This inhibits phospholipase A_2, which converts membrane phospholipids into arachidonic acid.

Further reading

Burgen AS. Targets of drug action. *Annu Rev Pharmacol Toxicol* 2000; 40: 401–416

Yamakura T, Bertaccini E, Trudell JR, Harris RA. Anaesthetics and ion channels: molecular models and sites of action. *Annu Rev Pharmacol Toxicol* 2001; 41: 23–51

4	Measures that can be taken to minimize central-venous catheter related infections

Definitions and criteria for diagnosis of central venous catheter-related infections vary. In general, however, two patterns are seen. Colonization refers to asymptomatic growth of organisms on the catheter, whereas infection associated with signs or symptoms is referred to as catheter-related bacteraemia (CRB). It is generally accepted that colonization precedes CRB but only a small fraction of colonized catheters become an infection problem.

Measures to decrease colonization and CRB include:

- *Selection of insertion site.* In order of decreasing infective complications, the commonly used sites are subclavian, internal jugular and femoral.
- *Subcutaneous tunnelling.* Although commonly performed there is little evidence to support this practice.
- *Insertion by an experienced operator.* Infection, like many complications, can be reduced by good technique.
- *Skin preparation.* Thorough skin cleansing with an appropriate agent such as 2% chlorhexidine in alcohol or povidone–iodine is essential.
- *Sterile technique.* Full aseptic precautions should be used, i.e. hat, mask, gown, gloves and a large drape.
- *Dressings.* No single dressing type seems to be superior. However, a sterile dressing should be applied and changed if it becomes damp, loose or soiled.
- *Duration of placement.* The longer a catheter remains in situ, the greater is the risk of infection. Catheters should be changed when clinically indicated. There is no evidence to support scheduled changes after predetermined intervals. New catheters should be inserted through a new puncture site. Some authorities recommend the old catheter being 'rewired' and replaced at that site and then changing the catheter if the old catheter tip is colonized.
- *Changing of fluid administration sets.* Infection risks increase as the integrity of the catheter/giving set complex is breached. Therefore unless clinically indicated the giving sets should not be changed more frequently than every 72 hours.
- *Catheter materials.* Most catheters are composed of polyurethane. This has a low infection rate similar to Teflon but is less likely to cause thrombophlebitis. Some catheters impregnated with antimicrobial agents have been shown to reduce infection, particularly those incorporating chlorhexidine and silver sulphadiazine or combinations of rifampicin and minocycline.

Further reading

Fraenkel DJ, Rickard C, Lipman J. Can we achieve consensus on central venous catheter-related infections? *Anaesth Intensive Care* 2000; 28: 475–490

Pearson MP. Guidelines for the prevention of intravascular catheter-related infections, 2002. http://www.cdc.gov/ncidod/hip/iv/iv.htm

5 What physiological processes involve α_2-adrenergic receptors? Outline the investigated and potential clinical uses for α_2-agonists

Physiological processes involving α_2-receptors:

- Sedation – located within the locus coeruleus.
- Analgesia – predominantly spinal and/or peripheral.
- Alteration of heart rate (bradycardic drive), decreased tachycardia and enhancement of bradycardia (vagomimetic).
- Vasoconstriction via sympatholysis *plus* vasodilation via smooth muscle receptors.
- Anti-shivering properties – basis unclear.
- Diuretic properties-basis unclear.

Clinical uses:

- Attenuation of a hyperdynamic profile (e.g. post-thermal injury).
- Sedation on intensive care.
- Reducing inhaled volatile anaesthesia requirements.
- Treatment of pain.
- Neuropathic.
- Intractable.
- Acute postoperative pain (especially post-Caesarean section).
- Decreasing incidence of postoperative shivering.
- Altering incidence of perioperative myocardial ischaemia.

Further reading

Eisenach JC, De Kock M, Klimscha W. Alpha(2)-adrenergic agonists for regional anesthesia: a clinical review of clonidine (1984–1995). *Anesthesiology* 1996; 85(3): 655–674

Khan ZP, Ferguson CN, Jones RM. Alpha-2 and imidazoline receptor agonists: their pharmacology and therapeutic role. *Anaesthesia* 1999; 54(2): 146–165

6 List the potential neurological complications arising from obstetric regional anaesthesia

1 Inflammatory.
   - Aseptic meningitis.
   - Bacterial meningitis.
   - Arachnoiditis.
   - Epidural abscess.
2 Dural puncture headache and complications.
3 Bleeding.
   - Spinal haematoma.
   - Cranial subdural haematoma.
4 Anterior spinal artery syndrome.

5 Cranial nerve palsies.
   • Trauma neuropathy.
   • Radiculopathy.
6 Maternal obstetric palsies.
   • Lumbosacral plexus injury.
   • Common peroneal neuropathy.
   • Femoral neuropathy.
   • Obturator neuropathy.
   • Meralgia paraesthetica.
   • Spinal cord infarction.

Further reading

Loo C, Dahlgreen G, Irestedt L. Neurological complications in obstetric epidural anaesthesia. *Int J Obstet Anaesth* 2000; 9: 99–124

7 The physiological roles of albumin

Maintenance of colloid oncotic pressure

In healthy subjects 80% of the normal colloid oncotic pressure is provided by albumin. This is due to a direct osmotic effect plus attractive electrostatic forces (the Gibbs–Donnan effect).

Transport function

Many endogenous substances are bound to albumin in plasma. These include long-chain fatty acids, bilirubin, haematin, bile acids, copper, zinc and folate. Many drugs, including non-steroidal anti-inflammatory drugs, warfarin, digoxin, frusemide, benzodiazepines and some penicillins, are also transported bound to albumin. Binding influences drug distribution, effect and elimination.

Metabolic function

Binding to albumin inactivates some compounds, such as disulfiram and certain antibiotics. Albumin is also involved in the metabolism of endogenous substances such as lipids and eicosanoids.

Acid–base function

Albumin is highly negatively charged, which makes it a very effective plasma buffer. It is responsible for approximately half of the anion gap.

Antioxidant function

It is likely that albumin efficiently scavenges oxygen free radicals, which have been implicated in many disease states.

Maintenance of microvascular integrity

Albumin may play a part in limiting increases in capillary permeability. The mechanism is unclear but appears to be shared by synthetic colloids.

Anticoagulant effects

Albumin seems to exert a heparin-like effect and may also inhibit platelet aggregation.

Further reading

Nicholson JP, Wolmarans MR, Park GR. The role of albumin in critical illness. *Br J Anaesth* 2000; 85: 599–610

8   The risks of anaesthetizing a premature infant

Prematurity is defined as birth prior to 37 weeks gestation. Approximately 7% of all such births are less than 2.5 kg and only 0.5% weigh less than 1 kg. The risks of anaesthetizing a premature neonate are such that unless the surgery is essential no child under 60 weeks of post-gestational age should undergo surgery. The main problems are:

1 *Apnoeic spells.* Oxygen consumption is higher relatively at about 7 ml kg^{-1} min^{-1}.
2 *Airway closure.* Reduced lung compliance and small airways predispose to airway closure and atectasis.
3 *Bradycardia.* Increased susceptibility to reflex bradycardia and hypotension may be a reflection of a mature parasympathetic system or an immature sympathetic system.
4 *Hypothermia.* Large surface area to weight ratio and lack of subcutaneous fat.
5 *Hypoglycaemia.*
6 *Pharmacology.* Neonates are sensitive to induction agents (reduced plasma protein binding) and muscle relaxants – atracurium is cleared a little faster. Opiates may exacerbate apnoeic problems.

The major risks are related to apnoeic spells, which may occur as late as 12 hours following surgery and in about 20–30% of healthy neonates. Centrally mediated apnoea is the most common cause, followed by obstruction. Prolonged observation is necessary as these episodes may be quite common in the postoperative period and respiratory stimulants may be necessary in some of these children. The risk of apnoea decreases with increasing gestational age and local anaesthetic techniques may reduce the risk of this complication. The problems may be exacerbated by anaemia, which is also common. The haemoglobin falls in the first 3 months so that paradoxically, as the problems of prematurity recede, the potential effects of anaemia increase.

Improved survival in very low birthweight infants has resulted in increased chronic respiratory problems in this population, so that a significant proportion of premature neonates have chronic lung disease and will require close observation for several days postoperatively because of poor oxygenation even without apnoeic periods.

There is increased interest in the use of regional techniques where possible.

Further reading

Crean PM. Anaesthesia for the premature infant. *Curr Anaesth Crit Care* 2000; 11: 245–249

Larsson BA. Pain management in neonates. *Acta Paediatr* 1999; 88(12): 1301–1310

9 The common causes and effects of hypomagnesaemia

The total body magnesium is about 25 g, largely in bone and teeth. The plasma level is normally 1.2–2.0 mmol 1^{-1}. It is protein bound and competes with calcium for binding sites. There is far more intracellular magnesium than extracellular and hence (in terms of movement in and out of the cell) it behaves like potassium or phosphate. Similarly plasma measurement does not necessarily reflect total body magnesium.

Magnesium is important in the function of many enzyme systems (e.g. creatine phosphokinase), protein synthesis and has a role at the neuromuscular junction, influencing the sensitivity to acetylcholine of the end-plate as well as the release of acetylcholine.

The commonest causes of low plasma magnesium are malabsorptive states, diarrhoea and hyperaldosteronism. Of these, diarrhoea is the most common.

Hypomagnesaemia may occur with hypokalaemia as its movement is to some extent linked with potassium. Problems that affect potassium such as diuretics or primary aldosteronism will also affect magnesium. It may be seen in diabetic ketoacidosis associated both with the diuresis and with the changing acid–base status. Likewise hypocalcaemia, which may occur in hypoparathyroidism, may concomitantly influence magnesium.

Muscle weakness, lethargy and depression are common symptoms. If the levels fall further, muscle fasciculations are seen and later tetany that is calcium resistant. Cerebral irritability and convulsions may occur. There may be psychiatric manifestations.

Patients with congestive heart failure are predisposed to magnesium deficit for many reasons, including neurohormonal activation, poor gastrointestinal absorption and drug therapy. Hypomagnesaemia is common in these patients and has been linked to an increased frequency of complex ventricular ectopy.

There is an association between cardiac irritability and magnesium with potential prolonging of the Q–T interval.

Further reading

Olerich MA, Rude RK. Should we supplement magnesium in critically ill patients? *New Horiz* 1994; 2(2): 186–192

Whang R, Hampton EM, Whang DD. Magnesium homeostasis and clinical disorders of magnesium deficiency. *Ann Pharmacother* 1994; 28(2): 220–226

10   Zopiclone

Zopiclone is a cyclopyrrolone hypnosedative. It has both sedative and anxiolytic properties. It is unrelated to the benzodiazepines. It potentiates γ-aminobutyric acid (GABA)-mediated neuronal inhibition.

Unlike the benzodiazepines it has a limited effect on normal sleep architecture, with very little rapid eye movement (REM) suppression. This may be due to it having a different site of action on the GABA–benzodiazepine receptor complex, where it appears to enhance chloride channel opening. It is very short acting, with an elimination half-life or about 3 hours. It is reputed to have a better spectrum of activity in terms of interfering with daytime function. In that respect zopiclone appeared to have somewhat better effects on daytime well-being than midazolam.

There is little evidence of risk of withdrawal reactions with therapeutic doses of zopiclone and dependency appears very low.

Further reading

Hajak G. A comparative assessment of the risks and benefits of zopiclone: a review of 15 years' clinical experience. *Drug Saf* 1999; 21(6): 457–469

Wadworth AN, McTavish D. Zopiclone: a review of its pharmacological properties and therapeutic efficacy as an hypnotic. *Drugs Aging* 1993; 3(5): 441–459

11   Factors that influence the passive diffusion of drugs across cell membranes

The body can be considered to consist of different aqueous compartments that are separated from each other by lipid membranes having varying degrees of specialization. Passive diffusion is only one of a variety of mechanisms by which drugs and other small molecules can traverse these membranes, but it is one of the more important in relation to pharmacokinetic mechanisms. The permeability coefficient of a drug relates to the number of molecules traversing a membrane of given area in a given time, when a concentration gradient for the drug exists across the membrane.

Two chemical factors contribute to the permeability coefficient, these being solubility and diffusivity. The main factor that determines the rate of transfer of a substance across a cell membrane is its lipid solubility, essentially because the cell membrane has high lipid content. Solubility is normally expressed as an oil/water partition coefficient. The higher the partition coefficient, the greater the drug's affinity for the lipid phase over the aqueous phase and so the more rapid its diffusion through the membrane.

Diffusivity relates to the ability of a drug to be mobile within the substance of a membrane and is expressed as a diffusion coefficient. This varies little between drugs, making the oil/water partition coefficient the more important variable. As the rate of diffusion is inversely proportional to the square root of molecular weight for small substances and the cubed root for large substances, it can be seen that molecular weight is a less important factor in determining diffusional transfer. As most drugs are either weak acids or bases, this means that they can exist in either ionized or unionized forms. The degree of ionization of such a drug will vary according to the environmental pH and the drug's pK_a as determined by the Henderson–Hasselbalch equation. Generally it is only the unionized species that is able to cross the cell membrane and this can give rise to ion trapping either side of a membrane which separates two aqueous environments of differing pH.

12 Perioperative care of patients' eyes

Damage to patients' eyes during surgery may not only be painful but also result in permanent damage. Awareness of the causes of damage is needed to prevent them. Direct injury can occur to the eye, and is often inflicted by the anaesthetist's fingers, watch strap and equipment post induction. Inhalational anaesthetic agents can be irritant to the eyes. In theatre the eye can be damaged during the application of surgical skin preparations or drapes. Postoperatively, vigilance must be maintained while the patient regains consciousness, as attempts to rub the eyes often involves the cannulated hand.

Exposure of the cornea, as well as direct damage, can result in corneal abrasions. Over 50% of patients fail to close their eyes completely during anaesthesia. If the period of exposure exceeds 1 hour, the incidence of corneal damage increases. Tear production decreases under general anaesthesia and the stability of the tear film also decreases.

Pressure effects can cause serious damage to the eye. Direct pressure on the globe can impair retinal blood flow, leading to ischaemia and possible blindness. Pressure from face masks can reduce choroidal blood flow and therefore ischaemia of the peripheral cornea. Raised venous pressure can result in corneal oedema.

To prevent damage, the anaesthetist needs to ensure that the patient's eyes are closed during the operative period, checking after repositioning. Simply taping the eyes is effective. The additional use of paraffin and water-based ointments does not decrease the occurrence of abrasions and the paraffin-based ointments may cause increased morbidity. The prone and lateral positions are the most common causes of ocular pressure injuries, and the anaesthetist must ensure that there is good venous drainage, no direct pressure on the globe and that the eyelid is closed. Ocular damage is often easily preventable and it is the anaesthetist's responsibility to remain aware of the problem.

Further reading

Roth S, Thisted RA, Erickson JP, Black S, Schreider BD. Eye injuries after nonocular surgery: a study of 60,965 anesthetics from 1988 to 1992. *Anesthesiology* 1996; 85(5): 1020–1027

Write short notes on the following topics. Do not miss out any questions and remember that there are only 3 hours in total to complete this paper.

1　The features and management of congenital diaphragmatic hernia
2　Aldosterone
3　Complications of radial artery cannulation
4　The null hypothesis, and outline errors associated with its use
5　The 'rotameter': how it works
6　Air embolism
7　Excitatory amino acid antagonists in neuroprotection
8　Positive end-expiratory pressure
9　The interpretation of liver function tests
10　Pulmonary and respiratory function in the elderly
11　Paravertebral analgesia
12　Inter-hospital transfer of trauma patients

1   The features and management of congenital diaphragmatic hernia

Congenital diaphragmatic hernia (CDH) occurs in 1:3600 live births when the fetal diaphragm develops leaving an opening between the thorax and the abdomen, allowing abdominal contents to enter the thoracic cavity.

The diaphragm forms during the eighth to tenth week of life, the left posterolateral segment between the lumbar and costal muscle fibres being the last to close. This is the site of 70–90% of herniations and has been termed the foramen of Bochdalek.

The midgut returns to the abdominal cavity during the tenth week and can enter the thorax when there is a defect in the diaphragm. Duodenal malrotations are commonly associated with CDH.

There is coexisting lung hypoplasia with a decrease in the number of airways and alveoli and a decrease in the number of pulmonary arteries. The arteries are abnormally distributed and there is an increase in the amount of smooth muscle found in the arterioles. Pulmonary hypertension is the result.

There remains some doubt whether the primary problem is abnormal development of the lung or of the diaphragm.

Features

CHD usually presents soon after delivery but may be delayed, particularly if the hernia is small. Antenatal diagnosis is increasingly common.

- There will be respiratory distress, mediastinal shift away from the side of the hernia, decreased breathing sounds and possible bowel sounds on the affected side. A scaphoid abdomen may indicate significant herniation. Gas-filled loops of bowel may be evident on chest X-ray.
- Pulmonary hypertension can cause right-to-left shunting through the foramen ovale and ductus arteriosus, resulting in refractory hypoxaemia.

Management

These neonates frequently require resuscitation and intensive care. If diagnosed antenatally the baby is usually delivered electively in an appropriate centre and intubated and ventilated immediately. This is to prevent distension of the stomach by gas, which risks further compromising ventilation.

Special attention is required to minimize the degree of pulmonary hypertension by ensuring adequate oxygenation and preventing respiratory and/or metabolic acidosis. Aggressive hyperventilation risks barotrauma, and on occasion sodium bicarbonate is used. Good sedation and the prevention of hypothermia and hypoglycaemia are also important.

Tolazoline, magnesium sulphate and nitric oxide have been used as pulmonary vasodilators.

The degree of pulmonary hypoplasia ultimately determines outcome and a period of stabilization before any surgery is an accepted management.

The role of extracorporeal membrane oxygenation for infants in whom maximal medical management has failed may offer the chance of survival, but has yet to be fully evaluated.

Surgery involves a transverse abdominal incision and either primary closure of the defect or the use of a patch to avoid any tension. A chest drain is not usually inserted, to allow fluid to accumulate in the space left by the hypoplastic lung.

Outcome

Overall survival is around 50% and is closely related to the degree of lung hypoplasia. The lungs of survivors will continue to grow, so that the long-term outlook is good. Small abnormalities of pulmonary function can be detected.

Further reading

Muratore CS, Wilson JM. Congenital diaphragmatic hernia: where are we and where do we go from here? *Semin Perinatol* 2000; 24(6): 418–428

Weber TR, Kountzman B, Dillon PA, Silen ML. Improved survival in congenital diaphragmatic hernia with evolving therapeutic strategies. *Arch Surg* 1998; 133(5): 498–503

2   Aldosterone

Aldosterone is the major mineralocorticoid hormone and is synthesized in the zona glomerulosa of the adrenal cortex. When secreted, its effect is to conserve sodium by increasing the reabsorption of Na^+ from the urine, sweat, saliva and gastric juice. In the renal tubules, Na^+ is exchanged for K^+ and, to a lesser extent, H^+. This results in acidic urine and the loss of K^+. Water retention occurs secondary to Na^+ reabsorption and so, as a consequence, aldosterone increases the extracellular fluid volume. These effects occur within 1 hour of its release and continue for several hours. At a cellular level, aldosterone diffuses across the cell membrane, where it binds to specific cytoplasmic receptors. This hormone–receptor complex then migrates into the nucleus, where it induces the synthesis of proteins involved in Na^+ and K^+ transport.

The release of aldosterone is stimulated by:

- The renin–angiotensin system.
- Hyponatraemia.
- Hyperkalaemia.
- Adrenocorticotrophic hormone (ACTH).

Of these, hypovolaemia is the most important. Hypovolaemia acts to increase aldosterone secretion via the renin–angiotensin system. Hyponatraemia and hyperkalaemia both have a direct effect in the zone glomerulosa. Hyponatraemia also acts to stimulate the renin–angiotensin system. Surgery, anxiety and stress all increase aldosterone production, as does increasing ACTH levels.

Atrial natriuretic peptide (ANP) inhibits renin as well as the responsiveness of adrenal gland to angiotensin II.

Hyperaldosteronism occurs when the adrenals secrete too much aldosterone with sodium retention. The result is also hypokalaemia, often with hypertension. The accompanying systems are vague and non-specific. They include muscle weakness, nocturia and tetany. Hypertension may be severe. Primary hyperaldosteronism, a rare cause of hypertension, is caused by hormone-secreting tumours of the adrenal cortex. Adrenal adenomas (Conn's syndrome) account for two-thirds of cases, while most of the rest are due to bilateral adrenal hyperplasia. Secondary hyperaldosteronism is much more common. It is seen in cirrhosis, heart failure, nephrosis, renal artery stenosis, accelerated hypertension and chronic diuretic therapy.

Spironolactone, a diuretic, is used in situations where there is oedema owing to secondary hyperaldosteronism. It acts as a competitive antagonist of aldosterone. Hypoaldosteronism is rare except as a component of primary adrenal cortical failure (Addison's disease).

3   Complications of radial arterial cannulation

Arterial cannulation is commonly performed to allow continual arterial pressure monitoring and easy access for sampling. The waveform allows both pressure measurement and a visual representation of pulsatile blood flow.

Complications involve:

- Disturbance of blood flow distant to the site of cannulation.
- Structural damage to the artery – aneurysm formation.
- Accidental injection of drugs or air with chemical irritation or embolism.
- Disconnection with bleeding.
- Infection.

Damped or ringing waveforms provide inaccurate measurements that may result in inappropriate intervention or failure of appropriate intervention.

In the presence of inadequate collateral flow, interruption of radial artery flow will result in ischaemia of the hand. Traditionally, an Allen's test is recommended to test for ulnar collateral circulation. Both radial and ulnar arteries are compressed, while the patient clenches their fist. On release of the ulnar artery there should be prompt return of colour to the hand. This provides some reassurance that collateral flow is adequate but it is not absolute. Flow distal to the site of cannulation may also be interrupted by embolism of atheromatous plaque or clot. Prevention of clot formation is aided by the use of Teflon cannulae and constant flushing of the system.

Structural damage such as intimal tears may occur, which can lead to aneurysm formation. Accidental injection of drugs into the arterial system can lead to major ischaemic problems within the hand owing to vascular spasm and drug precipitation.

Following accidental intra-arterial injection prompt treatment with vasodilators and sympathetic blockade is required to try and dilate the vessels, thus maintaining circulation. There is also the possibility of air entering the flushing system, which would also result in embolism. Accidental disconnections may occur on moving the patient; they should be obvious and easily corrected.

Further reading

Gillies IDS, Morgan M, Sykes MK et al. The nature and incidence of complications of peripheral arterial puncture. *Anaesthesia* 1979; 34(5): 506–9

Lee KL, Miller JG, Laitung G. Hand ischaemia following radial artery cannulation. *J Hand Surg [Br]* 1995; 20(4): 493–495

4 The null hypothesis, and outline errors associated with its use

In comparing different populations, two basic theories underpin tests of statistical significance.

The first is the null hypothesis, which theorizes that the groups do not differ in any way and that any observed differences must have arisen by chance. The second is the alternative hypothesis which holds that the groups come from different populations.

Significance testing is used to evaluate the probability that the null hypothesis should be rejected. It is possible to come to the wrong conclusion. There are two possible errors. In a type 1 error, the null hypothesis is rejected when it is, in fact, true: false positive. The chance of a type 1 error occurring is minimized by choosing a p-value of less than 0.05 ($p < 0.05$). The lower the level of probability at which an outcome is thought to be significant, the less is the chance of a type 1 error.

A type 2 error occurs when the null hypothesis is accepted when it is, in fact, false:false negative. The probability that we do not commit this type of error is called the power of a test. In general, increasing the sample size will increase the power of a test. Ideally, a comparative study between different populations should be designed to minimize both these types of errors. In reality this can be difficult.

5 The 'rotameter': how it works

A rotameter is a device which is used to measure gas flow. This is a rotating bobbin type of flow-meter that is simple and easy to use, yet is sufficiently accurate for clinical use. It is a constant-pressure, variable-orifice device. The tube varies in diameter along its length and the taper is wider at the top. Some have a double taper. The higher the rotating bobbin is lifted by the gas flow, the wider the gap around it becomes. The pressure across the bobbin remains constant because it has a constant weight, but the area of the annular orifice increases with higher gas flows.

The gas flow in the lower part of the tube depends on viscosity, because it acts as a tubular orifice which leads to laminar flow through the orifice. As the gap becomes wider, and the orifice becomes more annular, turbulence is more likely and the flow is more dependent on the density of the gas. The tubes are calibrated at 1 atmosphere pressure and room temperature and for a specific gas only. This is because of the differential effects of the viscosity and density as the flows alter.

The accuracy of these devices is of the order of ±5%. Factors involved in the accuracy of the device are as follows:

- An increase in atmospheric pressure will cause the flow-meter to over-read.
- Gases with increased viscosity will over-read at low flows.
- Gases with a greater density will over-read at high flows.
- The effects of changes in ambient temperature are limited.

The tubes must be vertical. As the rotation of the bobbin is likely to generate static electricity, there must be conducting material to remove this or the bobbin will stick. Therefore the tubes may be coated internally with a conduction material, often a thin film of gold, and earthed at both ends, again often with a fine gold band.

Potential problems of the oxygen flow-meter include the delivery of hypoxic mixtures if:

- there is leakage either at the top end of the tube or distal to the flow meter.
- The oxygen flow-meter is upstream of other flow-meters for other gases such as nitrous oxide.

Back-pressure from ventilators will not alter flow rate but might alter the value reading in the flow-meter. The bobbin is fluted or notched to make it spin and reduce the likelihood of it sticking, but this may still occur if the bobbin becomes dirty or contaminated.

6   Air embolism

Air embolism occurs if:

- Air is entrained into the circulation.
- There is iatrogenic insufflation of air or other gas (laparoscopy).
- Air is introduced via venous access lines or intra-arterially.
- Via an extracorporeal circulation.

The factors that influence the importance of air embolism are:

- The volume.
- Rate of introduction.
- Presence of a right–left shunt, e.g. patent foramen ovale.

Whenever an open vein is above the level of the heart there is a risk of air embolism developing. Thus in both practice and theory air embolism can develop even when the patient is horizontal. The anaesthetist should be aware that this complication is still possible even though the risk is much lower than if the patient is in the sitting position. As air accumulates in both the right ventricle and in the pulmonary circulation it will both reduce cardiac output and some regions of pulmonary blood flow.

The capnograph will detect a fall in end-tidal CO_2 when venous air embolism takes place, as the cardiac output falls and as air is trapped in the pulmonary vascular bed. There is an increase in effective physiological dead space due to the large number of alveoli which are no longer being perfused. Thus, as ventilation does not alter there will be a fall in CO_2 excreted. Paradoxical embolism is undoubtedly more lethal than venous embolism as small volumes of air in either the coronary or cerebral arteries can cause sudden death. The development of paradoxical embolism has been recorded in patients with normal cardiac anatomy, although the risk is greater in those who have a patent foramen ovale.

Signs of air embolism include the following:

- Rapid entrainment may make hissing noise.
- Air in the right ventricle produces a 'mill-wheel' murmur.
- Cyanosis.
- Hypotension.

Diagnosis is made in the following ways:

- Clinically.
- Oesophageal stethoscope.
- Doppler ultrasonic flow detector on praecordium.
- Monitor end-tidal CO_2.

Treatment:

- Prevent further air entry. Head-down posture; flood the wound and open area with saline; apply gentle neck compression to partially occlude the neck veins and cause venous engorgement.
- Left lateral position to hold air away from entrance to the pulmonary artery.
- Give oxygen to help remove any nitrous oxide (nitrous oxide will increase gas volume in the blood).
- Infuse fluid to increase right filling pressure and wash out froth.
- Try and aspirate air via central line.

Further reading

Muth CM, Shank ES. Gas embolism. *N Engl J Med* 2000; 342(7): 476–482

Williamson JA, Webb RK, Russell WJ, Runciman WB. The Australian Incident Monitoring Study. Air embolism: an analysis of 2000 incident reports 1993. *Anaesth Intensive Care* 1993; 21(5): 638–641

7 Excitatory amino acid antagonists in neuroprotection

L-Glutamate is an excitatory amino acid widely distributed in the central nervous system and is responsible for the majority of excitatory signals in fast-conducting sensory input and interneurone pathways via glutamate-sensitive cation channels. Excess release of L-glutamate causes neuronal damage and it is proposed that damage caused by a wide variety of neuronal insults may be due, in part, to excessive release of glutamate and overaction of postsynaptic receptors. Glutamate-gated cation channels fall into two groups, AMPA and NMDA, according to the synthetic agonist to which they respond. The NMDA receptor plays a key role in excitotoxicity, probably because of a high permeability to calcium, which is a known mediator of cell damage. Unusually, the NMDA receptor is inactivated by Mg^{2+} under resting conditions. This NMDA receptor also contains a glycine site, which is another potential site of NMDA antagonist action.

Selective NMDA and AMPA receptor antagonists have been shown to be protective against neuronal damage in both in-vitro and in-vivo animal studies. Animal evidence suggests better neuronal protection with focal ischaemia using NMDA antagonists but better protection in global ischaemia with AMPA antagonists. Clinical evidence is limited and trials are ongoing.

Psychotomimetic and cardiovascular side effects may limit the use of many agents. However, glycine antagonists and intravenous magnesium are better tolerated.

Further reading

Lees GJ. Pharmacology of AMPA/kainate receptor ligands and their therapeutic potential in neurological and psychiatric disorders. *Drugs* 2000; 59(1): 33–78

Meldrum BS. Glutamate as a neurotransmitter in the brain: review of physiology and pathology. *J Nutr* 2000; 130(4S Suppl): 1007S–1015S

Petrie RX, Reid IC, Stewart CA. The N-methyl-D-aspartate receptor, synaptic plasticity, and depressive disorder: a critical review. *Pharmacol Ther* 2000; 87(1): 11–25

8 Positive end-expiratory pressure

Positive end-expiratory pressure (PEEP) is used to improve oxygenation in ventilated patients. The application of PEEP to the lungs of a ventilated patient helps to prevent atelectasis of alveoli during the expiratory phase of the ventilatory cycle and may also help to recruit alveoli that have previously collapsed. This improves the functional residual capacity of the lung, promoting improved arterial oxygenation for a given inspired oxygen concentration. Alveoli that do collapse owing to zero or inadequate PEEP may remain collapsed and are then no longer available for gas exchange. Instead, these collapsed alveoli act as areas of shunt or ventilation–perfusion mismatch, which have the adverse effect of causing arterial hypoxia.

PEEP has beneficial effects on oxygenation, but these may be at the expense of cardiovascular compromise. The additional of PEEP causes a decrease in venous return to the heart owing to positive pressure in the thorax throughout the ventilatory cycle. A decrease in venous return will decrease the cardiac output. The positive pressure in the thorax increases the afterload of the right ventricle, impairing ejection and so causing greater diastolic volume. This causes right ventricular distension, promoting septal shift, which in turn will impair the filling of the left ventricle and so decrease cardiac output. The heart is also subjected to positive intrathoracic pressure at all times, which decreases its compliance and therefore impairs filling, decreasing cardiac output. Other effects of PEEP include decreased renal perfusion, decreased gut perfusion, hepatic congestion and the possibility of increased intracranial pressure. The beneficial effects of PEEP on oxygenation, therefore, need to be titrated against its possible deleterious effects on the cardiovascular system.

Further reading

Kloot TE, Blanch L, Melynne-Youngblood A et al. Recruitment maneuvers in three experimental models of acute lung injury: effect on lung volume and gas exchange. *Am J Respir Crit Care Med* 2000; 161(5): 1485–1494

Lu Q, Rouby JJ. Measurement of pressure–volume curves in patients on mechanical ventilation: methods and significance. *Crit Care* 2000; 4(2): 91–100

Pelosi P, Goldner M, McKibben A et al. Recruitment and derecruitment during acute respiratory failure: an experimental study. *Am J Respir Crit Care Med* 2001; 164(1): 122–130

9 | The interpretation of liver function tests

The liver function tests (LFTs) generally include:

• Plasma total bilirubin	2–17 μmol l^{-1}
• Aspartate aminotransferase	10–40 U l^{-1}
• Alanine aminotransferase	5–40 U l^{-1}
• Alkaline phosphatase	25–115 U l^{-1}
• Albumin	35–45 g l^{-1}

The normal range may vary between laboratories. LFTs in general reflect either the consequences of the liver being unable to perform adequately or the measurement of enzymes being released from liver cells. The former will represent either under-performance of the liver or excess production of the substrate that exceeds the liver's capacity to clear the material, e.g. bilirubin. The latter is confounded by similar enzymes being released from other cells and from the observation that the quantity in the plasma does not necessarily indicate rate of release or ongoing release. It does not provide a dynamic indicator of liver function. Tests that attempt to look at dynamic function do exist but are difficult to use in practical clinical terms.

Bilirubin is a breakdown product of haemoglobin formed in the reticuloendothelial system. It is insoluble in water in its unconjugated form and is initially loosely bound to albumin. In the hepatocytes it undergoes conjugation with glucuronide, making it water soluble, and is excreted in the bile. In the gut bilirubin is converted to urobilinogen, some of which is absorbed to be re-excreted by the liver or to be excreted into the urine by the kidneys. An increase of unconjugated bilirubin is usually caused by an increase of its production owing to haemolysis, or inability to conjugate it because of an enzyme defect such as in Gilbert's syndrome. These forms of hyperbilirubinaemia are usually associated with normal results in the other LFTs. Urinary urobilinogen may be raised in haemolysis as the liver's ability to excrete becomes overloaded. Conjugated hyperbilirubinaemia occurs when there are functional hepatocytes but obstruction to the flow of bile. It can be caused by intrinsic liver disease or biliary tree disease. Conjugated hyperbilirubinaemia is associated with urinary urobilinogen, unless there is complete biliary obstruction.

The aminotransferase level represents hepatocyte integrity. Any damage to or death of hepatocytes results in an increase in aminotransferase levels, as these cytosol enzymes leak out of the liver. The more acute the damage, the greater the rise of these enzymes, which may reach 100 times their normal value in acute viral infections or acute hepatitis due to drugs.

Chronic infection leads to chronic low-level enzyme elevation. The aminotransferase enzymes can also become markedly raised as a result of hypotension.

Alkaline phosphatase is found in almost all tissues. Cholestasis induces hepatic alkaline phosphatase synthesis, the enzyme then leaking from the biliary tree into the blood. The highest levels are found in obstructive cholestasis, levels being raised to a lesser degree in hepatocellular disease. As alkaline phosphatase arises in many different tissues, it can be raised in a variety of conditions. For this reason, a raised level with no other abnormal LFT should be viewed suspiciously and an extrahepatic source of alkaline phosphatase sought.

Lactate dehydrogenase (LDH) is not often measured. It catalyses the conversion of lactate to and from pyruvate, so it also has a high concentration in heart, lung, skeletal muscle, kidney, brain and erythrocytes. It is non-specific and is now often used as a marker of lung injury.

Albumin is synthesized by the liver and its level will be reduced in chronic hepatocellular disease. It should be remembered, however, that many other disease processes can cause a low albumin level. Similarly the prothrombin index may reflect the ability of the liver to synthesise clotting factors, but this is also influenced by other factors that affect coagulation.

Further reading

Ayling RM. Pitfalls in the interpretation of common biochemical tests. *Postgrad Med J* 2000; 76(893): 129–32; quiz 132,169

Dufour DR, Lott JA, Nolte FS, Gretch DR, Koff RS, Seeff LB. Diagnosis and monitoring of hepatic injury. II. Recommendations for use of laboratory tests in screening, diagnosis, and monitoring. *Clin Chem* 2000; 46(12): 2050–2068

10 Pulmonary and respiratory function in the elderly

The lungs change with age and the most obvious change affects pulmonary elasticity. The elastin content in the lung decreases and the fibrous connective tissue increases; this leads to a progressive loss of lung elastic recoil. The ageing lung becomes more compliant, but the small airways are also more likely to collapse and increases in anatomical dead space occur. There is a thinning of the inter-alveolar walls, leading to loss of surface area and breakdown of septae. This causes an increase in alveolar dead space. Chest wall compliance decreases because an increasing thoracic curvature and calcification of costochondral joints make the chest wall more rigid. The balance of these changes is that despite maintenance of 'normal' total pulmonary compliance with ageing, there are falls in the expiratory reserve volume because of an increase in residual volume. One of the effects of reduced elasticity is to increase the closing volume and, by the age of 65 years, this begins to encroach into tidal ventilation when lying down. As this progressively deteriorates with advancing age there is an increasing alveolar–arterial gradient for oxygen and falls in the arterial oxygen tension. The fibrosis and calcification of the chest wall lead to a reduction in forced expiratory volume in 1 second, and also limit the elderly patient's maximal breathing capacity and increase their work of breathing.

Their control of breathing is also less robust. The elderly have a reduction in their ventilatory response to hypoxia and hypercapnia and during sleep they have an increased incidence of episodic obstruction leading to apnoeas. When they have significant cardiovascular as well as pulmonary changes they also have an increased incidence of periodic breathing. Both of these control problems make them more likely to have apnoea and airway obstruction perioperatively.

They have reduced sensitivity to irritants and may not respond to airway contamination, especially when there are trace amounts of anaesthetic agents present. Their upper airway tone progressively falls with age (hence the increased incidence of snoring) and combined with the frequent loss of dentition may lead to difficulties maintaining a patent airway during induction, maintenance and recovery from anaesthesia. The elderly are believed to be more sensitive to the respiratory depressive side effects of the opiate analgesic drugs, but whether this is a 'real' observation or a reflection of increased bioavailability of these drugs has not been clearly answered.

Further reading

Bhatia PK, Bhandari SC, Tulsiani KL, Kumar Y. End-tidal oxygraphy and safe duration of apnoea in young adults and elderly patients. *Anaesthesia* 1997; 52(2): 175–178

Zaugg M, Lucchinetti E. Respiratory function in the elderly. *Anesthesiol Clin North Am* 2000; 18(1): 47–58, vi

11   Paravertebral analgesia

Paravertebral analgesia is a useful technique for surgical procedures of the abdomen and thorax, particularly where the afferent input is predominantly one-sided, e.g. open cholecystectomy, nephrectomy, mastectomy and thoracotomy. It has been in use for most of the twentieth century although interest in its use has been variable.

The standard technique requires placing the patient in a lateral position with the side to be blocked uppermost. Intravenous access and appropriate monitoring are required for this aseptic procedure. The spinous process is palpated and 2–3 cm lateral to the spinous process a short bevelled spinal needle or a Tuohy needle (if a catheter is required) is advanced at right angles to the skin, in all planes. Once the needle has struck the transverse process then it is 'walked' over the top of the process using a loss-of-resistance technique with air or saline. Test aspiration to ensure there is no blood or cerebrospinal fluid. Following successful placement without aspiration of blood and cerebrospinal fluid, a catheter can be introduced or local anaesthetic can be used. Typically, a volume of 15 ml may spread over five dermatomes in an average adult. An overall failure rate of 10% is usual.

Complications include:

- Hypotension.
- Vascular puncture.
- Pleural puncture.
- Pneumothorax.
- Rarely, evidence of distant spread such as Horner's syndrome, epidural block and total spinal.

There are few contraindications except local sepsis or empyema. Local tumour and allergy to the local anaesthetics are rare. Anatomical abnormalities may make the procedure difficult and serious complications more likely.

Further reading

Lonqvist PA, MacKenzie J, Soni AK, Conacher ID. Paravertebral blockade: failure rate and complications. *Anaesthesia* 1995; 50(9): 813–815

Richardson J, Lonnqvist PA. Thoracic paravertebral block. *Br J Anaesth* 1998; 81(2): 230–238

12   Inter-hospital transfer of trauma patients

Inter-hospital transfer is frequently necessary. Good communication is essential prior to transfer. The referring doctor should give a clear history and a summary of the findings and treatment given. The receiving doctor should be available for advice. All notes, X-rays, results and any available cross-matched blood should accompany the patient. Prior to departure resuscitation should be complete. Ideally a specialist transfer team should be used but failing that the accompanying persons must be competent at airway, fluid and resuscitation management.

A – Airway and cervical spine

There should be a low tolerance to the insertion of an endotracheal tube, because as with many practical procedures this will be difficult en route. If there is any possibility of cervical injury the cervical spine should be adequately immobilized with a collar. Placement of a gastric tube will be beneficial in reducing the risk of aspiration.

B – Breathing

Intubated patients should be mechanically ventilated and once adequate sedation is assured it is beneficial to paralyse. Monitoring with capnography, pulse oximetry and invasive haemodynamic lines is recommended. Consider giving 100% O_2. For long journeys it is advisable to calculate how much oxygen is required as the ambulance supply is finite. As with intubation there should be a lower tolerance to the insertion of chest drains and these should be attached to a Heimlich valve. A urine bag will hold any fluids from the drain.

C – Circulation

Haemorrhage should have been controlled, but adequate fluid resuscitation will need to continue and should be prepared for. Adequate venous access is mandatory and arterial access is advisable for monitoring. These should be visible to prevent inadvertent exsanguination.

D – Disability

Sedation is a form of treatment as well as being humane. Continuous infusions provide better cardiovascular stability. Controlled ventilation for neurotrauma transfers is mandatory with a Glasgow Coma Scale score of less than 8.

E – Everything else

Empty the urine bag. Splint the fractures. Cover the patient. Keep warm. The transfer should be by an experienced doctor with a trained assistant. Monitoring should follow minimum guidelines with continuous observation, ECG, SpO_2, blood pressure (invasive preferably), ventilation disconnect alarm. Capnography can provide useful information.

Further reading

Bellingan G, Olivier T, Batson S, Webb A. Comparison of a specialist retrieval team with current United Kingdom practice for the transport of critically ill patients. *Intensive Care Med* 2000; 26(6): 740–744

In this section, ten clinical scenarios are described. The responses to the scenarios may be found following this section and are there as a guideline. Clearly in many of these several different responses are possible and this should engender debate.

This section of clinical scenarios should ideally be used after passing the written papers, or as a focus for discussion within a group of candidates at the same stage of preparation for the exam. They are a series of clinical cases or vignettes that should be used to test presentation skills and to display knowledge, judgement and safety in a viva setting. Ideally two 'examiners' should be used, one to ask the question and the other to observe both the questioner and the 'candidate'. The aim has to be to encourage and support the 'candidate' to cover the ground effectively, not to display superiority in knowing the answers. If an area of profound ignorance is discovered it should be left. There is nothing to gain from trying to define the limits of lack of knowledge – it is simply destructive. Far more is to be gained by moving to a scenario where the candidate can perform better.

Remember that the answers provided are the views of experts, but equally valid points may be raised and covered.

The choice of scenarios should be of a group of two or three giving a broad field of topics. They should be reviewed in advance by the 'examiners' and they should take alternate turns in observing and questioning. The observer should write down the answers given and any good or poor examples of examining.

Debriefing is as important as the viva itself, the areas that should be covered include:

The 'candidate'

Appropriate sense of urgency – is this a life-threatening case? Is there a sense of this in the answer? Does the management conform to that expected from such serious problems?

Is the answer structured? Random comments show a clear lack of preparation and often of poor knowledge. Prompting may help the nervous but will only unmask ignorance of a topic.

Is the presentation clear? Video recording is an easy and effective method to demonstrate both the good and the bad habits of candidates. Talking too quietly to deaf, elderly examiners is a bad as adding irrelevant noises to disguise the thought processes – the umm syndrome.

Is there demonstration of balance? The scenarios in the examination are seldom simple, and a clear conflict of interest may occur – these are not built into all of these scenarios but they could be added if necessary to expand on the testing of a candidate's judgement. Usually the safety issues take precedence; all others are open to debate.

The 'examiner'

Were the scenarios presented clearly? Write them down and print them out. Practise reading them, and learn the answers – or at least be able to see them. Examiners who get the question right and the answers wrong can be as destructive as those who aggressively seek out weaknesses.

Were they supportive? Laughing at the candidate or falling asleep are thought to be poor form. Failing to observe the non-verbal communication from the candidate will often result in the loss of opportunities to get the best from the candidate.

Were they consistent? It is very easy to examine on areas of personal interest but this has two hazards. The first is of being too expert and failing to identify a safe and reasonable level of knowledge. The second is to turn the viva into a tutorial. It is often easier to be consistent with areas where the examiner knowledge base is simply good.

Finally, review the whole process. The aim of examining is to gain insight into how questions can be phrased to elicit the appropriate answer and just how hard it can be to ask apparently simple questions. The act of practising from both sides will improve technique and the ability to understand what the 'real' examiner wants on the day of the examination.

Consider the following clinical scenarios as a presentation at a viva and review your answers to display judgement and prioritization. Remember that a display of knowledge without clinical interpretation is unlikely to impress the examiners, and that these answers are indicative only. You may disagree and have differing but equally acceptable answers.

Scenario 1

An ASA 1, 35-year-old woman is scheduled for a laparoscopic cholecystectomy. General anaesthesia is induced with propofol and fentanyl, and muscle relaxation is provided by rocuronium 0.5 mg kg^{-1}. She receives intermittent positive-pressure ventilation via a tracheal tube. Soon after induction of pneumoperitoneum the pulmonary inflation pressure is noted to rise from 18 cmH$_2$O to 35 cmH$_2$O.

1   What is your differential diagnosis?
    Despite additional muscle relaxants the problem persists. The patient develops a tachycardia of 120 bpm. The end-tidal carbon dioxide concentration rises to 6.5 kPa then suddenly falls to 2 kPa. Peripheral oxygen saturation falls to 88%.
2   What is the most likely diagnosis now?
3   How could you confirm this diagnosis?
4   How do you manage this patient?
5   What is the prognosis?

Scenario 2

A 10-year-old boy weighing 80 kg has been investigated by respiratory physicians for sleep apnoea. Continuous pulse oximetry while he is asleep has shown that his SaO$_2$ falls intermittently to 64%. He is noted to have large tonsils and has been referred to an ENT surgeon for consideration for tonsillectomy. The surgeon decides that tonsillectomy is appropriate.

When seen preoperatively, he is a very obese child with poor venous access. Examination is otherwise normal. An ECG has been carried out by a perceptive house surgeon and shows prominent R waves in V$_{1-3}$, and an inverted T wave in V$_3$.

Consider the following points:

1   What is the likely reason for sleep apnoea?
2   Why did the perceptive house surgeon do an ECG?
3   What do the changes in the ECG represent?
4   What is the reason for the cardiovascular condition which causes the ECG changes?

5 Would any other simple investigations confirm this cardiovascular state?
6 Consider the premedication for this child.
7 Would you give a neuromuscular blocking agent?
8 Are there increased cardiac risks?
9 Where should he be managed postoperatively?
10 Should he be ventilated postoperatively?

Scenario 3

A 40-year-old woman presents to have a hysterectomy for menorrhagia. She is an insulin-dependent diabetic who was diagnosed about 30 years ago. She injects 12 units of neutral insulin (Actrapid) morning and evening and 12 units of insulin zinc suspension (Monotard) in the morning. She is generally symptomatically well. She has had several uneventful anaesthetics in the past.

Consider the following points:

1 What preoperative investigations are mandatory?
2 Are there any other investigations or tests you would carry out preoperatively?
3 Is there any test which would indicate the stability of her diabetes in the recent past?
4 What alterations to her insulin regimen would you make in the perioperative period?
5 Would you perform a preoperative chest X-ray?
6 What is likely to happen to the blood glucose level during the operation?
7 What premedication would you prescribe?
8 Is there any contraindication to a regional block for this procedure?
9 Are any special precautions necessary at induction of general anaesthesia?
10 What maintenance intravenous fluid would you use during the operation? Are there any that should be particularly avoided in this case?
11 During the operation, considerable variations in blood pressure are encountered. What may these be particularly due to in this case?
12 Are variations in blood pressure during the operation any more potentially harmful in this patient than in a non-diabetic patient?
13 What special precautions, if any, should be taken in the recovery room?
14 Is there any contraindication to patient-controlled analgesia in this patient?
15 Is this patient more at risk from deep vein thrombosis than a non-diabetic patient who is otherwise identical in her general medical state?
16 What is the incidence of diabetes in the population who require a surgical operation?
17 Do diabetic patients require surgery more frequently than non-diabetics?

18 What percentage of diabetics have an affected relative?

19 Do diabetics have an increased perioperative mortality compared with non-diabetics?

20 What is the commonest single cause of death in diabetics?

Scenario 4

A man aged 70 years who suffers from hypertension, angina on moderate exertion and chronic obstructive airways disease needs a transurethral prostatectomy. His usual medication includes captopril. A single reading of his blood pressure on admission is 180/100 mmHg.

Consider the following points about his management:

1 Which of the following preoperative tests should be performed: ECG, chest X-ray, lung function tests, arterial blood gases?

2 Does his blood pressure require further treatment?

3 What premedication, if any, would you use?

4 Would you prescribe any prophylaxis against perioperative cardiac ischaemia? If so, what?

5 Assuming no absolute contraindication, would you use general epidural or spinal anaesthesia?

6 If you used general anaesthesia would you use spontaneous ventilation or controlled ventilation? Which volatile agent would you use, and why?

7 If you used spinal anaesthesia, which gauge needle would you use, for preference?

8 What is the lowest systolic blood pressure you would regard as safe?

9 Would you prescribe oxygen therapy during the first postoperative night?

10 Is there any contraindication to opioid analgesia postoperatively?

Scenario 5

A 79-year-old woman has been admitted and a provisional diagnosis of perforated bowel has been made. An urgent laparotomy is required. On visiting the patient on the ward, you find her clinically dehydrated, peripherally shut down, with a regular heart rate of 110 bpm and a blood pressure of 100/80 mmHg. She is confused and in pain and no useful medical history can be obtained, although she has a bottle of frusemide tablets in her possession. No investigations are available yet.

Consider the following points:

1 Which of the following investigations should be performed?

   • Haemoglobin.
   • Blood urea.

- Serum creatinine.
- Serum electrolytes.
- ECG.
- Chest X-ray.

2 Would you order cross-matched blood?

3 Would you postpone surgery until she was rehydrated?

4 Would you set up a central venous line preoperatively?

5 What induction agent would you use?

6 What neuromuscular blocking drugs would you use?

7 Would you set up an epidural block for postoperative analgesia?

8 Is this patient at risk of a deep vein thrombosis?

The surgeon finds a perforated colonic diverticulum, with faecal peritonitis. The surgeon mobilizes the bowel with difficulty, performs a limited resection and brings out a defunctioning colostomy. The procedure takes 2 hours. You have given 3 litres of intravenous fluid (crystalloid and colloid) to maintain the central venous pressure (CVP):

1 At the end would you reverse the neuromuscular blockade and attempt to extubate the trachea?

2 Would the patient's condition and other factors justify taking the last ICU bed in the hospital?

Scenario 6

A 25-year-old man is scheduled for extraction of impacted wisdom teeth under general anaesthesia. His preoperative assessment is unremarkable and he appears to be a particularly fit man, involved in many sports and physical activity. Induction of anaesthesia is with thiopentone, suxamethonium, nasotracheal tube and pharyngeal pack and maintenance with nitrous oxide, oxygen and isoflurane with spontaneous respiration. During the operation he appears to be lightly anaesthetized, as shown by hyperventilation and muscle movements. The surgeon notes that the jaw muscles appear rigid. At the end of the operation, the patient's HbO_2 saturation on the pulse oximeter is 91%.

Consider the following points:

1 Is the anaesthetic technique appropriate to the operation?

2 What is the most significant reason for the hyperventilation and apparent light anaesthesia?

3 What monitoring would most readily reveal the reason for this complication?

4 What treatment should be initiated for this condition?

5 What later complications may occur?

6 What other anaesthetic agents or drugs may produce this condition?

7   What is the incidence of this complication in the general population?

8   How might this complication have been predicted preoperatively?

9   What advice would you give to the patient about future anaesthetics?

10 What help organizations exist in the UK for susceptible patients and their relatives?

Scenario 7

A 19-year-old man is brought to the accident and emergency department of your district general hospital having been involved in a road traffic accident in which he was the front seat passenger. On first assessment, he is semi-conscious, opens his eyes on command, but is restless and aggressive. His speech is inappropriate. He says he is in severe pain from his right thigh, which is swollen and distorted. Neurological examination at this stage, apart from the deterioration in consciousness, is normal.

While in the radiology department he becomes less aggressive and then unrousable except to painful stimulus, which results in localized response. The radiographs show a fracture of the shaft of the right femur and a small depressed fracture of the skull in the right frontoparietal region.

An intravenous infusion has been established by the paramedics at the site of the accident and he has so far received 1 litre of Hartmann's solution and 500 ml of hetastarch.

Consider the following points:

1   Does he need further investigations? If so, what are they?

2   Does he need transfer to a specialist neurosurgical unit?

3   What should be done before he is transferred?

4   What are the indications for transfer of a patient who has had a head injury to a specialist unit?

5   If he is to be transferred, what staff should accompany him and should he be observed en route?

6   What scoring system is commonly used in head injury patients? What is his score (i) on admission (ii) in the radiology department?

7   The CT scan shows a large extradural haematoma. Should this be evacuated through a burr-hole before transfer?

8   Should an intracranial monitoring system be introduced before transfer?

9   On arrival in the neurosurgical unit, the first priority will be for which of these?
    (a) Repeat CT scan to assess the development of the haematoma.
    (b) Controlled ventilation in ICU to reduce brain bulk.
    (c) Craniotomy.

10 Prognosis – what to tell the family.

Scenario 8

A 9-month-old infant is admitted for repair of a U-shaped midline cleft of her palate. She weighs 5 kg. Her mother reports she has been a poor feeder since birth, failing to gain weight and requiring a number of hospital admissions with chest infections possibly following choking episodes with feeds. On examination, jaw recession is noticeable. Palpation of the lower border of the mandible feels bowed. The child has no other gross dysmorphic features. Cardiovascular system examination and an ECG are normal. Observation of respiration at rest reveals intermittent intercostal recession. Lateral X-ray of the jaw is reported as showing mandibular hypoplasia with marked shortening of the ramus and a concave depression in the lower border of the body of the mandible.

1 What is the underlying condition and why is its identification important?
2 Describe any premedication you would prescribe and what instructions you would give to the ward relating to feeding on the morning of operation.
3 Describe how you would undertake induction of anaesthesia in this patient.

Scenario 9

A 20-year-old man is admitted with a 12-hour history of pain in the right testicle. He is in considerable pain and has vomited repeatedly in the last few hours. He was diagnosed as having diabetes mellitus 10 years ago and is currently on 15 units of soluble insulin twice a day.

On examination the testicle is swollen and tender. A presumptive diagnosis of torsion of the testicle has been made and exploratory surgery is planned. His blood glucose level is 28 mmol l^{-1} and his urine, which is scanty, is reported as '+++ ketones'.

Consider the following points:

1 How urgent is the operation?
2 What should be done to control his diabetes?
3 Are any other investigations necessary at this stage?
4 Are any complications of diabetes likely to be relevant during this operation?
5 It is appropriate to give him opioids for analgesia before the operation?
6 How should his diabetes be managed during the operation?
7 What anaesthetic technique would you use?
8 What complications is this patient especially prone to in the immediate (first hour) postoperative period?
9 What other surgical procedure will be carried out at the time of operation?
10 Is he likely to have severe postoperative pain?

A 5-year-old boy is admitted with a 1-day history of fever and increasing shortness of breath. He has been given ampicillin syrup by his general practitioner, but his condition has worsened in the last 2 hours. He has no pain but has a sore throat.

On examination he is restless, febrile and has marked noisy dyspnoea with supraclavicular and intercostal recession. He is drooling saliva and crying hoarsely. His temperature is 38.5°C, pulse 160 bpm and respiratory rate 30 breaths min^{-1}. His SaO$_2$ while breathing air is 93%.

Consider the following points:

1 What is the likely diagnosis?
2 Would a chest X-ray be helpful at this point?
3 Would any other investigations be appropriate at this point?
4 Which of the following actions would be appropriate now (choose more than one if appropriate):
   (a) Continue with antibiotics, humidified oxygen and observation on the open paediatric ward.
   (b) Inset an arterial line for blood gases.
   (c) Admit to ICU for observation.
   (d) Intubate under general anaesthesia after inhalation induction with oxygen and halothane and observations of the larynx.
5 On direct laryngoscopy, you see a red cherry-like swollen epiglottis and oedematous tissues around the laryngeal inlet. The cords are not visible. What manoeuvre might help you to determine where the glottis is?
6 Having successfully intubated the child, would you put him on a ventilator?
7 What would you use to sedate the child?
8 For how long is he likely to need intubation?
9 What organism is most likely to be responsible for this condition?
10 What antibiotic would be appropriate for this condition?

Scenario 1

1 Differential diagnosis:

- Inadequate muscle relaxation.
- Kinking of the tracheal tube.
- Endobronchial intubation.
- Bronchospasm.
- Pneumothorax.
- Gas embolism.

2 What is the most likely diagnosis?
The pattern of the rise of the end-tidal CO_2 followed by a sudden fall is characteristic of pulmonary embolism. However, end-tidal CO_2 concentration often rises during pneumoperitoneum and any sudden fall in cardiac output may produce these changes.

3 How could you confirm this diagnosis?
Diagnosis depends on recognizing the presence of gas in the right side of the heart or on its consequences.

- Detection of gas emboli.
- Precordial or oesophageal Doppler.
- Aspiration of gas or foam from the central venous catheter.
- It is unlikely that a central catheter or Doppler probe are in place for a laparoscopic cholecystectomy.
- Presence of a characteristic mill-wheel murmur.
- Capnography changes are discussed above.

Consequences of embolization:

- Rise in pulmonary artery pressure.
- Rise in central venous pressure.
- Tachycardia/arrhythmias.
- Hypoxaemia.
- ECG changes of right heart strain.
- Pulmonary oedema.

Other signs:

- Blood on aspiration from Verres needle.
- Pulsation of flow-meter pressure gauge.
- Absence or disappearance of abdominal distension despite sufficient volumes of insufflated gas.

4 How do you manage this patient?

- Cease insufflation and release pneumoperitoneum.
- Place patient in head-down left lateral position (Durant's position).
- 100 % oxygen – will improve oxygenation.
- hyperventilation to increase CO_2 elimination.
- Insertion of a central venous or pulmonary artery catheter to aspirate the gas if the above measures fail to improve the situation.

- Cardiopulmonary resuscitation.
- In extreme cases cardiopulmonary bypass has been used.

5 What is the prognosis?

Due to the high solubility of CO_2 in blood the prognosis is good if treatment is instituted early. However, fatalities do occur.

Further reading

Palmon SC, Moore LE, Lundberg J, Toung T. Venous air embolism: a review. *J Clin Anesth* 1997; 9(3): 251–257

Weissman A, Kol S, Peretz BA. Gas embolism in obstetrics and gynecology: a review. *J Reprod Med* 1996; 41(2): 103–111

Scenario 2

1 The cause of sleep apnoea is not known for certain but it is common in obese males. It is thought that collapse of pharyngeal tissues may cause obstruction during slow wave sleep. Enlarged tonsils are not usually thought to be an important factor but enlarged adenoids will cause mouth breathing, which is associated sleep apnoea.

2 Obstructive sleep apnoea is associated with right heart strain.

3 The ECG changes represent right ventricular hypertrophy. The inverted T wave in V_3 suggests that this is severe.

4 The right heart strain is the result of pulmonary hypertension, caused by hypoxic vasoconstriction.

5 Pulmonary artery and lateral chest radiographs would confirm right-sided cardiac enlargement. An echocardiograph would assess the degree of functional impairment.

6 Difficult! Heavy sedation might result in sleep apnoea. At this age, he is probably amenable to encouragement by the anaesthetist, obviating the need for premedication. Venous access is likely to be difficult and EMLA cream should be applied freely over a number of veins.

7 Although some anaesthetists would ventilate all children for tonsillectomy, most allow spontaneous ventilation. This would be quite inappropriate in his case because of his obesity and because of the need for rapid return of reflexes.

8 No increased risk. According to Goldman (1978) there is no increased risk from right heart failure unless there is a third heart sound (gallop rhythm) and/or jugular venous congestion.

9 Although the removal of his tonsils is supposed to have improved his airway, there are still risks of obstruction and underventilation due to his obesity. Management on the paediatric ward is inappropriate. Therefore he should at least be in the high-dependency unit (HDU). Unfortunately many hospitals do not have an HDU, so the ICU is the only option.

10 Ventilation is not mandatory, but he will need very careful monitoring and regular assessment. An arterial line should have been sited during the operation to allow regular blood gas (PaO_2 and $PaCO_2$) monitoring, and continuous pulse oximetry is essential.

Further reading

Goldman L, Caldera DL, Southwick FS, Nussbaum SR, Murray B, O'Malley TA, Gorol AH, Caplan CH, Nolan J, Burke DS, Krogstad D, Carabello B, Slater EE. Cardiac risk factors and complications in non cardiac surgery. *Medicine (Baltimore)* 1978; 57(4): 357–370

Loadsman JA, Hillman DR. Anaesthesia and sleep apnoea. *Br J Anaesth* 2001; 86(2): 254–266

Warwick JP, Mason DG. Obstructive sleep apnoea syndrome in children. *Anaesthesia* 1998; 53(6): 571–579

Scenario 3

1 Investigations:
   (a) Haemoglobin estimation, because she has menorrhagia and therefore may have iron deficiency anaemia. An acceptable lower limit is a matter of debate. A high proportion of the world's population exist in reasonable health with a haemoglobin level in single figures, and increased 2,3-DPG levels in the blood permit compensation in the increased carriage of oxygen. Most conservative Western anaesthetists would prefer a level of 9 g dl^{-1} or above, especially as there may be underlying ischaemic heart disease.
   (b) Blood urea and creatinine levels, because long-standing diabetes is often accompanied by impairment of renal function.
   (c) Blood glucose level. This should be taken at the same time of day as the proposed operation to give an indication of adequacy of control with the perioperative regimen. At the same time, evidence of ketosis should be sought. If present it is an absolute indication to postpone the operation and seek the opinion of a diabetologist as she will need assessment of the stability of her diabetes prior to elective surgery.
   (d) There are other tests than can be done (see below) but whether they contribute is debatable.

2 (a) An ECG is important because of the high incidence of ischaemic heart disease in diabetics. Whether a resting ECG is helpful is doubtful unless the ischaemia is considerable. The purists would say that a physical stress ECG or even an echocardiogram would give better information.
   (b) Others are referred to below.

3 An estimation of the glycosylated haemoglobin gives an indication of the stability of the blood glucose over the preceding few weeks, a level below 10% of total haemoglobin being satisfactory.

4 There are numerous regimens for the management of insulin therapy in the perioperative period. What is certain is that the regimen she is on now

would make it difficult to manage her diabetes during this time. Most anaesthetists would stop her present regimen on the day of operation and convert to a flexible control based on continuous infusion of 10% dextrose and a variable infusion of short-acting neutral insulin (Actrapid or similar), with 1-hourly monitoring of blood glucose levels and 3-hourly checks on serum potassium levels (since the regimen drives K^+ into the cells, producing plasma hypokalaemia). See the quoted reference at the end of this section for practical details. This regimen should be continued during the operation and into the postoperative period until she is taking a normal diet and is mobile. There is a tendency to relax the regimen postoperatively which must be resisted, since at this time she is at particular risk because of hyperosmolarity and dehydration causing venous thrombosis and pain, resulting in adrenergic antagonism of insulin.

5 The benefits are difficult to assess and usually it will contribute very little. There is an increased incidence of pulmonary tuberculosis in diabetics but it is very low and does not justify an X-ray. If she has not had a chest X-ray recently then it may provide a baseline if problems were to develop.

6 The adrenergic and adrenocorticoid response to surgery will antagonize the effects of insulin and cause a rise in blood glucose. This can be attenuated by adequate intraoperative analgesia, which should be used liberally. Some anaesthetics, such as ketamine, cause a greater rise in blood glucose than others – this would be an unusual technique to use in this case.

7 Premedication for anxiolysis. There is an increased likelihood of gastric stasis in this patient, as a result of autonomic (vagal) neuropathy, which would make one consider the use of preventative measures for the effects of gastric aspiration at induction. Metoclopramide does not antagonize gastric stasis due to vagal neuropathy. Ranitidine, with cricoid pressure at induction, would be prudent.

8 There are no contraindications to regional anaesthesia. Diabetics are more prone to infection and the aseptic technique you always use for your regional block is especially important, of course.

9 There are several special considerations prior to surgery:
   (a) Check the blood glucose to ensure that she is not hypoglycaemic at this time.
   (b) Gastric stasis is a risk due to vagal neuropathy, so some might perform a rapid-sequence induction.
   (c) Systemic autonomic neuropathy may result in hypotension at induction, particularly when controlled ventilation is started, especially if the patient is hypovolaemic as a result of your preoperative regimen. Have colloid fluids ± vasopressors ready.
   (d) Many long-standing diabetics have proliferative retinopathy and a hypertensive response to intubation may precipitate a vitreous haemorrhage. A generous dose of alfentanil and/or lignocaine will therefore be important just before intubation.
   (e) There may be occult ischaemic heart disease, even if the ECG is normal.

10 Fluid management is an issue. Glucose, although being given as part of the diabetic control, cannot be used in increased volume as this will require additional insulin. Classically Hartmann's was avoided because of the lactate

component, which is metabolized to glucose, but on current perioperative regimens this should not be a problem – nor is the lactate itself. The patient will require maintenance fluid and 0.9% sodium chloride is best unless the operation is exceedingly long. The volumes of glucose solution should be borne in mind when prescribing other maintenance fluid.

11 Intraoperative blood pressure variations may be due to;
   (a) Hypovolaemia as a result of preoperative fluid restriction.
   (b) Sympathetic neuropathy. This is very likely in a patient who has been diabetic for this length of time. An experienced diabetologist has expressed the opinion that any patient who has been insulin-dependent for more than 20 years is certain to have autonomic neuropathy. Colloid and vasopressors should be ready.

12 Detrimental effects from blood pressure variation. Many long-standing diabetics are vulnerable to renal insults such as hypotension. Those with perioperative periods of hypotension are more likely to develop renal failure postoperatively.

13 In the recovery room there are potential problems additional to those normally encountered in the immediate postoperative period:
   (a) Gastric stasis, leading to regurgitation of gastric contents into the lungs.
   (b) There is an increased incidence of cardiorespiratory arrest, presumably due to autonomic neuropathy.
   (c) Hypoglycaemia.

14 Patient-controlled analgesia. The adequacy of analgesia is important in maintaining stable control of her diabetes.

15 While there are plenty of reasons why an insulin-dependent diabetic should have a high risk of venous thrombosis, including obesity, hyperosmolar state and postoperative immobility, these appear to carry no greater risk than in equivalent non-diabetics. She is still at risk, though, and prophylactic measures (anti-embolic stockings, low-dose heparin, early mobility) are essential.

16 In the UK, about 3% of the surgical population are diabetic and this figure is increasing.

17 Diabetics are more likely to require medical interventions generally. This is because of the complications of diabetes, which include infections, arterial insufficiency, ophthalmic complications, cardiac surgery for ischaemic heart disease and renal problems.

18 There is a familial component to diabetes and 20% have an affected relative.

19 Theoretically, given the potential problems that a long-standing diabetic might have and the tendency to life-threatening complications, mortality should be higher. At least one controlled study, however, failed to show increased mortality.

20 The commonest cause of death is ischaemic heart disease.

Further reading

Ali MJ, Davison P, Pickett W, Ali NS. ACC/AHA guidelines as predictors of postoperative cardiac outcomes. *Can J Anaesth* 2000; 47(1): 10–19

Horton JN. Anaesthesia and diabetes. In: Nimmo WS, Rowbotham DJ, Smith G (eds). *Anaesthesia*. Blackwell Scientific, Oxford, 1994: 1077–1090

McAnulty GR, Robertshaw HJ, Hall GM. Anaesthetic management of patients with diabetes mellitus. *Br J Anaesth* 2000; 85(1): 80–90

Scherpereel PA, Tavernier B. Perioperative care of diabetic patients. *Eur J Anaesthesiol* 2001; 18(5): 277–294

Story DA, Aldridge J. Diabetes, blood glucose and preoperative evaluation. *Anaesth Intensive Care* 2000; 28(1): 110

Scenario 4

1 Preoperative tests might include ECG, chest X-ray, lung function tests and arterial blood gases. Each of them would reveal some aspect of his disease. None would be likely to reveal additional information, but each would provide a baseline against which postoperative changes can be assessed.

2 Should his blood pressure have additional treatment? No. There is evidence that hypertension, controlled by drugs, is satisfactory if the diastolic is below 110 mmHg. If there is doubt about this, further intervention should only be made after confirmation from at least two further readings of his blood pressure, at 4-hourly intervals.

3 Premedication? Explanation to reassure him and to assess his mental attitude.

4 Although many anaesthetists would use glyceryl trinitrate transdermal patches, there is little evidence that they affect outcome. They probably make everyone feel better, though.

5 Although outcome is probably not related to the method of anaesthesia, spinal anaesthesia would be the most popular choice. There is evidence that bleeding during prostatectomy is less when a regional block is used. Epidural anaesthesia is often technically difficult in the elderly and has no advantages over spinal anaesthesia.

6 If a general anaesthetic, controlled ventilation is to be preferred. The lithotomy position reduces vital capacity and the straining of spontaneous ventilation is likely to increase bleeding and prolong the procedure. The choice of volatile is interesting. Some might suggest isoflurane but this should be avoided as there is some evidence of 'coronary steal' which may precipitate myocardial ischaemia. Others would not consider this a specific contraindication. Most anaesthetists avoid halothane in adults, although the incidence of hepatocellular damage is much lower in the elderly.

7 Anaesthetists seem to take pride in using finer and finer needles for spinal blocks. The gauge of needle is relatively unimportant in this patient, compared to the parturient women. A 26-gauge needle would be difficult to introduce in this elderly patient and a 32-gauge almost impossible. The most important aspect of spinal anesthesia is ensuring a good block and then it is a compromise between needle gauge versus certainty of placement.

8 As a rule of thumb, a fall in blood pressure of about 33% would be tolerated without trouble. It is of course the diastolic pressure that decides the coronary blood flow.

9 Postoperative oxygen therapy should be prescribed, if possible, for the first three nights as this is the time when perioperative myocardial ischaemia is most likely to occur.

10 Are opioids contraindicated? No. Analgesia is important in this patient as pain will result in vasoconstriction and increase the likelihood of myocardial ischaemia.

Further reading

Reeves MD, Myles PS Does anaesthetic technique affect the outcome after transurethral resection of the prostate? *BJU Int* 1999; 84(9): 982–986

Windsor A, French GW, Sear JW, Foex P, Millett SV, Howell SJ. Silent myocardial ischaemia in patients undergoing transurethral prostatectomy: a study to evaluate risk scoring and anaesthetic technique with outcome. *Anaesthesia* 1996; 51(8): 728–732

Scenario 5

1 Haemoglobin, urea creatinine electrolytes, ECG and chest x-ray: all would confirm what is already known, with the exception of the chest X-ray, which some would say is irrelevant and unnecessary. In this case, in an elderly confused patient this would provide a baseline and an indication of whether aspiration, collapse or consolidation was present. Given the lack of clinical information the examination may well be complemented by the tests to indicate underlying disease, e.g. chronic renal failure, ischaemic heart disease, chronic airways disease. The value of the remaining investigations is in their guide to progress as treatment proceeds.

2 Cross-matching is probably unnecessary for the proposed operation, unless the haemoglobin is already very low, but serum should be sent to the blood bank for 'group and hold'.

3 Would you delay surgery to resuscitate? No. She requires urgent surgery to control the likely peritonitis, which is potentially lethal in this age group. But fluids should be given rapidly under CVP control, simultaneously with surgery. Colloids can be used but adequate fluid is needed.

4 Resuscitation of a dehydrated patient under these circumstances can be achieved easily and well without a CVP but it would facilitate management and might prevent fluid overload from rapid fluid administration. In dehydrated patients simple observation of the neck veins is an under-utilized clinical resource.

5 Avoidance of cardiovascular instability is the main intent. Etomidate has the advantage of cardiovascular stability. Ketamine would be many anaesthetists' choice. Judicious dosage of thiopentone!

6 Muscle relaxant: suxamethonium for a rapid sequence of induction (check that there is no hyperkalaemia first) and a cardiovascularly stable drug such as *cis*-atracurium for maintenance.

7 The role of an epidural – none, although this is controversial (see references). It is a potentially very hazardous procedure in a dehydrated septicaemic

patient. It would be difficult to be sure that the circulating blood volume had been restored and severe hypotension would be a significant risk. There is also probable bacteraemia.

8   This patient is definitely at risk of deep vein thrombosis. Dehydration, immobility and age are all risk factors. Low-dose heparin is essential in this case.

Following the case the decision of how she should be managed needs to be made. This will depend to some extent on the surgical findings, the ease of resuscitation and the cardiovascular stability throughout the case. Ideally she should be ventilated until cardiovascularly stable and rehydrated.

The issue of ICU admission is always difficult and must be determined on the factors prevailing at the time. These will include state of health prior to this event and the presence of other chronic disease factors:

- Magnitude of this event and impact in terms of stability during and in the initial postoperative phase.
- Recoverability from this event, which will take the above factors into account. The likelihood of returning to a state of well-being.
- The patient's own wishes if these can be determined.

These are a few of the factors that need to be considered.

Further reading

Elliott TB, Yego S, Irvin TT. Five-year audit of the acute complications of diverticular disease. *Br J Surg* 1997; 84(4): 535–539

Khan AL, Ah-See AK, Crofts TJ, Heys SD, Eremin O. Surgical management of the septic complications of diverticular disease. *Ann R Coll Surg Engl* 1995; 77(1): 16–20

Spackman DR, McLeod AD, Prineas SN, Leach RM, Reynolds F. Effect of epidural blockade on indicators of splanchnic perfusion and gut function in critically ill patients with peritonitis: a randomised comparison of epidural bupivacaine with systemic morphine. *Intensive Care Med* 2000; 26(11): 1638–1645

Scenario 6

1   Tracheal intubation is necessary. If spontaneous respiration is to be used, suxamethonium is a valuable aid to intubation, but it has a number of disadvantages, including muscle pains and a trigger effect on malignant hyperthermia. Many anaesthetists would use a non-depolarizing neuromuscular blocking agent and ventilate the patient's lungs throughout the operation. Isoflurane is a reasonable agent to use. Previously halothane had advantages, including smooth anaesthesia and relatively low cost, but is avoided (possibly unjustifiably) because of its common propensity to cause arrhythmias and its rare propensity to hepatitis and to trigger malignant hyperthermia. The more recent agents, sevoflurane or desflurane, are suitable alternative anaesthetics, especially if day care is planned.

2 Apart from the obvious reason, that the patient is not having enough anaesthetic, the possibility of malignant hyperthermia (MH) must be considered in this patient.

3 The best early indication of MH is an inappropriate rise in end-tidal CO_2 as a result of increased metabolic rate. Temperature rise is suggestive but is a late sign.

4 Stop the anaesthetic. Give oxygen only. Give dantrolene $2-10$ mg kg^{-1} i.v., plus supportive therapy for fluid loss, renal failure, hyperkalaemia and hypoxia. All theatres should have an MH management protocol, with a box of appropriate drugs in an identified place as part of their emergency protocols.

5 MH complications. Progressive acidosis, rising PCO_2 and falling PO_2. Hyperkalaemia. Clinical deterioration with tachycardia, hyperpnoea and arrhythmias. Later myoglobinuria leading to renal failure. Potentially cerebral hypoxia and myocardial failure.

6 The commonest trigger agents are halothane and suxamethonium. Other agents have also been implicated but it is noticeable that the incidence of this condition appears to have fallen since the use of suxamethonium and halothane has diminished with the availability of alternative agents.

7 Incidence is reportedly, between 1:6000 and 1:20 000. It appears to be less common in children and the elderly. Mortality appears to have fallen to about 25%, possibly due to earlier detection by intraoperative CO_2 and SaO_2 monitoring.

8 MH occurs, paradoxically and tragically, in fit young patients, particularly in athletes. Whether there is a connection between muscle development and MH is unproven. There is a fairly strong inherited tendency and, because of its dominant inheritance, siblings and children of known cases of MH carry a 50% probability of inheritance of susceptibility.

9 It is important to emphasize that susceptibility does not preclude general anaesthesia if it is required. There are plenty of non-trigger anaesthetic agents including thiopentone, morphine and the new neuromuscular blocking agents, and no patient need fear denial of general anaesthesia provided the anaesthetist is aware of the patient's susceptibility.

10 Help organizations. Of several, two are:

- Medicalert, 12 Bridge Wharf, 156 Caledonian Road, London N1 9UU, UK.
- Malignant Hyperpyrexia Society, 11 Gorse Close, Newthorpe, Notts NG162E, UK.

Further reading

Harriman DG, Malignant hyperthermia myopathy: a critical review. *Br J Anaesth* 1998; 60(3): 309

Morgan PG, Sedensky MM. A review of molecular genetics for the anaesthetist. *Eur J Anaesthesiol* 1995; 12(3): 221–247

Strazis KP, Fox AW. Malignant hyperthermia: a review of published cases. *Anesth Analg* 1993; 77(2): 297–304

1 Investigations needed: A CT or MRI scan of his head and cervical spine are essential to identify intracranial bleeding and an unstable cervical spine. Other than that, investigations should be as few as possible to avoid delay in active treatment, which is urgent.

2 Transfer is needed. Indications for transfer of head-injured patients are given in item 4 below.

3 Immediate management:
   (i)   Volume replacement of blood loss from his fractured femur and other injuries. This is essential as hypovolaemia and raised intracranial pressure will reduce his cerebral arterial perfusion pressure.
   (ii) Airway control and oxygenation, which initially will be by face mask, but as soon as his conscious level deteriorates he should be intubated and controlled ventilation instituted. This should be done by an experienced anaesthetist after administration of a bolus of alfentanil to suppress the adrenergic response to intubation and a full paralysing dose of a neuromuscular blocking agent to permit cough-free intubation. Following intubation he should be ventilated with full neuromuscular blockade to lower the arterial CO_2 tension and analgesia (alfentanil or similar) should be given as appropriate, to avoid adrenergic responses to painful stimuli.
   (iii) Monitoring of arterial blood pressure (preferably by direct arterial line), pulse, ECG, end-tidal CO_2 and SaO_2 should be established and continued until and during transfer to the neurosurgical unit. All hospitals which receive accident victims should have portable monitoring facilities available. Suitable units, such as the Propak and the HP Nomad, are available.

4 Indications for transfer of a head injured patient to a specialist neurosurgical unit include:
   (a) Deterioration in neurological status.
   (b) Skull fracture, unless asymptomatic. Depressed fractures must be transferred, regardless of neurological status.
   (c) Focal neurological signs.
   (d) Unconsciousness.
   (e) Confusion lasting more than 6 hours.

5 Transfer personnel: a doctor (usually with anaesthetic experience) capable of managing controlled ventilation, fluid replacement and cardiovascular instability. This requires experience and is often left to inadequately trained juniors. In one author's unit, the policy is to use the senior registrar on call, thus providing an experienced doctor while leaving the junior doctor resident in the hospital, covered by the consultant on call. Other units will not have this range of staff available, but should have contingency plans to provide an experienced doctor while not leaving the base hospital without adequate cover.

6 The Glasgow Coma Scale (GCS). This is an adequate overall scoring system but takes no account of important localizing signs, such as unilateral pupil dilatation, which should also be recorded. On admission, this man's GCS was

11 (eye opening 3, motor response 5, verbal response 3). Later, he has a GCS of 7 (eye opening 1, motor response 5, verbal response 1). This deterioration further supports urgent transfer to a neurosurgical unit.

7   A burr-hole has no role here. It wastes time and most general hospitals and surgeons will not be equipped for it.

8   Intracrania pressure monitoring monitoring system prior to transfer: although readily introduced systems are available, there is little additional information that can be gained at this stage and another delay is introduced.

9   The priority on arrival at the neurosurgical centre, the CT scan having already been done, is to evacuate the haematoma. Thus craniotomy is the priority, although a short period in ICU may be necessary if the theatre is not immediately available. Any delay reduces the chances of full recovery, however, and this case is in the NCEPOD category of 'emergency'.

10   Be guarded in the prognosis as the outcome is variable and unpredictable.

Further reading

Fearnside M, McDougall P. Moderate head injury: a system of neurotrauma care. *Aust NZ J Surg* 1998; 68(1): 58–64

Murray GD, Teasdale GM, Braakman R et al. The European Brain Injury Consortium survey of head injuries. *Acta Neurochir (Wien)* 1999; 141(3): 223–236

Lannoo E, Van Rietvelde F, Colardyn F, Lemmerling M, Vandekerckhove T, Jannes C, De Soete G. Early predictors of mortality and morbidity after severe closed head injury. *J Neurotrauma* 2000; 17(5): 403–414

Roberts I, Schierhout G, Alderson P. Absence of evidence for the effectiveness of five interventions routinely used in the intensive care management of severe head injury: a systematic review. *J Neurol Neurosurg Psychiatry* 1998; 65(5): 729–733

Scenario 8

1   The infant has Stickler syndrome, one of the syndromes lumped together as Pierre–Robin sequence. Stickler syndrome is an autosomal dominant disorder with characteristic ophthalmological and orofacial features, deafness and arthritis. Abnormalities of vitreous gel architecture are a pathognomonic feature, usually associated with myopia and a risk of retinal detachment. Children with Stickler syndrome typically have a flat midface with depressed nasal bridge, short nose, anteverted nares and micrognathia. These features can become less pronounced with age. Midline clefting, if present, ranges in severity from a cleft of the soft palate to Pierre–Robin sequence. Identification is important because:

- Intubation is likely to be difficult.
- Stickler syndrome carries the risk of blindness at an early age, potentially avoidable by early recognition and treatment.
- Identification of the underlying condition allows genetic advice to be given.

2 Premedication: atropine 20 μg kg^{-1} intramuscularly 30 minutes preoperatively. Sedatives will be avoided in view of the history of upper airway obstruction at rest. It is now clearly shown that clear fluids may be safely given up to 2 hours preoperatively.

3 An inhalational induction using halothane in 100% oxygen is advised, as visualization of the larynx may be difficult. A range of oral and nasal airways, bougies, laryngoscope blades and a fibre-optic laryngoscope should be available. An SpO$_2$ monitor should be in place on induction, with ECG and intermittent blood pressure recorder added as soon as tolerated by the infant.

Further reading

Lynch M, Underwood S. Pulmonary oedema following relief of upper airway obstruction in the Pierre–Robin syndrome: a consequence of early palatal repair? *Br J Anaesth* 1991; 66(3): 391–393

Wheatley RS, Stainthorp SF. Intubation of a one-day-old baby with the Pierre–Robin syndrome via a laryngeal mask. *Anaesthesia* 1994; 49(8): 733

Scenario 9

1 The operation is urgent. Even though he is of an age where epididymo-orchitis is more likely, the differential diagnosis is difficult and good surgical practice, backed by medicolegal precedent, requires urgent exploratory surgery to save the testis if it is ischaemic.

2 He has diabetic ketoacidosis as a result of his illness and in particular the repeated vomiting. This should not be tackled by the inexperienced and the help of an experienced diabetologist should be sought. The fundamental problems with diabetic ketoacidosis are dehydration from an osmotic, sugar diuresis. This produces a salt and water deficit but with excessive water loss and the loss is from all compartments. The acidosis is both from inappropriate metabolic pathways, due to insulin lack, but may also be due to poor perfusion from dehydration. The mandatory osmotic diuresis will have depleted potassium and the acidosis will have resulted in a potassium shift extracellularly along with phosphate. There will be a body deficit of both of these, which will become manifest as the insulin and the correction of the acidosis results in intracellular movement of these electrolytes.

He is inevitably dehydrated and needs urgent and adequate rehydration with either crystalloids, saline or colloids. It is not the type of fluid that is important, just that he has a replete intravascular volume. He will need insulin given under careful control by frequent blood glucose and potassium estimations. This will probably include intravenous insulin infusions starting at 5 units.h^{-1}. Much later, once his blood sugar is less than 12 mmol l^{-1} he will need fluid containing dextrose, such as 5% dextrose, which will both replace his water deficit and prevent hypoglycaemia if his sugar falls too far.

Electrolytes: he will need potassium supplements and may also need some phosphate. Any infection present should be treated. These problems must be balanced against the pressing need to get him to theatre within 1 hour.

Cooperation between senior colleagues is essential and the anaesthetist should be fully involved from the start. He may have to accept a less than optimally controlled patient.

3 Apart from the investigations relating to his ketoacidosis (pH, blood gases, potassium, sodium, urea, creatinine, glucose), probably not. A white cell count may help in the differential diagnosis but should not alter the plan to explore the testis.

4 He is a relatively long-standing diabetic so the possibility of autonomic neuropathy should be watched for. This may affect the sympathetic system (postural hypotension or hypotension in response to raised intrathoracic pressure during IPPV) or the parasympathetic system (gastric stasis at induction, made worse by pain and by opioids for pain relief). Diabetic retinopathy is a possibility so sharp rises in blood pressure at intubation should be avoided in case of retinal detachment. A generous dose of alfentanil 30 seconds before intubation is the best way to prevent this.

5 Opioids are not contraindicated. He will need adequate analgesia.

6 Assuming he is under control before induction, the best way to manage his diabetes perioperatively is to continue the insulin and fluid infusions and to cross over to an infusion of 5% dextrose as the glucose falls below 12 mmol l^{-1}. This may be of the order of 1 litre per 6 hours and a separate infusion of insulin 1–3 units per hour. Potassium should be checked every hour and potassium chloride added to the dextrose as necessary. This can be continued into the postoperative period until he is taking a normal diet.

7 The best thing would be a balanced anaesthetic technique following a rapid-sequence induction. This would ensure rapid recovery and avoidance of late complications on the ward when he had passed from the anaesthetist's immediate care.

8 These patients are prone to stop breathing in the immediate postoperative period. The reason is unclear but may relate to parasympathetic neuropathy. Recovery ward staff should be alerted to this possibility.

9 It is usual to carry out a fixation of the contralateral testis since both are prone to torsion. This adds to the operation time and may catch the anaesthetist out if he thinks the operation is complete when the affected testis has been dealt with.

10 He will probably have a measure of residual analgesia from the operative period. He should be assessed for need at the time. He may be more comfortable than he was preoperatively but he will still need analgesia.

Further reading

Delaney MF, Zisman A, Kettyle WM. Diabetic ketoacidosis and hyperglycemic hyperosmolar nonketotic syndrome. *Endocrinol Metab Clin North Am* 2000; 29(4): 683–705

Magee MF, Bhatt BA. Management of decompensated diabetes: diabetic ketoacidosis and hyperglycemic hyperosmolar syndrome. *Crit Care Clin* 2001; 17(1): 75–106

1 Diagnosis: acute epiglottis. The short history, noisy breathing and drooling of saliva are characteristic and distinguish the condition from acute laryngotracheobronchitis, which has a longer history and is not characterized by drooling of saliva.

2 A chest X-ray would be of no value and would waste valuable time. This child requires urgent intervention.

3 No other investigations are necessary at this time; routine blood count, etc. can be done later.

4 Appropriate actions would include:

- Intubate under general anaesthesia after inhalation induction with oxygen and halothane and observations of the larynx.
- Continue with antibiotics, humidified oxygen and observation on the open paediatric ward? *No*. This child's condition, especially the saturation of 93%, indicates that urgent intervention is required. He could develop complete respiratory obstruction at any time.
- Insert an arterial line for blood gases? *No*. A waste of valuable time and probably almost impossible in this restless child. An arterial line will be needed later, though, for monitoring of ventilation.
- Admit to ICU for observation? Possibly yes, for several reasons. Firstly, there are people on the unit with the skills to assess his airway and intervene when necessary. Secondly, the unit is staffed adequately for continuous observation. Thirdly, control of the airway by tracheal intubation can be carried out in ideal conditions. Lastly, the child is almost certain to end up on the ICU anyway.
- In fact the child needs *intubation, not ICU*.
- Anaesthetic technique: preferably an inhalational technique.
- Suxamethonium should not be given until the airway has been established and intubation and ventilation are possible. Halothane or sevoflurane, with its ability to induce anaesthesia smoothly, is ideal and will produce muscle relaxation fairly quickly to facilitate laryngoscopy. Because of its propensity for causing dysrhythmias and bradycardia, the ECG should be monitored.

5 A bubble of expired air coming through the oedematous mass may give a clue where the glottis is. This can be facilitated by pressing sharply on the chest.

6 Although there is a vogue for awake management of these children, the risk of losing the airway is significant. It is also a short-lived condition so that within hours it may be resolving. It is safer to sedate and ventilate the child than run the risk of potential extubation. A wide range of drugs can be used.

7 Traditionally, chloral $0.1-0.2$ g kg^{-1} has been used for sedation. Propofol is probably best avoided because of reports of hyperlipidaemia in children given infusions over a long time.

8 The child may need intubation for 2–3 days. 'Trial of extubation' should be carried out cautiously, with careful observation during the following few hours. Extubation should not be attempted in the evening or at night when

fewer staff are likely to be around. A useful sign that he is ready for extubation is the development of a leak around the tracheal tube as the laryngeal oedema diminishes.

9 The organism responsible is *Haemophilus influenzae*.

10 The antibiotic of choice is ampicillin or chloramphenicol.

Further reading

Cox PN. Current management of laryngotracheobronchitis, bacterial tracheitis and epiglottitis. *Intensive Care World* 1993; 10(1): 8–12

Consider the following clinical scenarios as a presentation at a viva and review your answers to display judgement and prioritization. Remember that a display of knowledge without clinical interpretation is unlikely to impress the examiners, and that these answers are indicative only. You may disagree and have differing but equally acceptable answers.

Scenario 1

A 75-year-old man has been admitted with a 2-hour history of increasing abdominal pain. On abdominal examination he has a large pulsatile tender swelling in the midline, which on bedside ultrasound scan is shown to be an expanding abdominal aortic aneurysm. He is alert and responsive. His blood pressure is 100/75 mmHg, pulse 88 bpm. Clinical examination of cardiovascular and respiratory systems is otherwise normal. He says he is very fit, he cycles 10 km on most days and plays golf every weekend. He is not on any drug therapy.

Consider the following points:

1. How urgent is the operation? What is the NCEPOD classification of the degree of urgency of this operation?
2. Is operation justified in his case?
3. What monitoring would you establish before inducing anaesthesia?
4. In addition to stored bank blood, what other blood products and in what quantity should be requested before the operation?
5. When the aorta is cross-clamped by the surgeon, what actions would you take?
6. What actions would you take when the cross-clamp is released?
7. In additional to replacement of blood loss, there is a need for fluid replacement from losses into the 'third space' (in this case, retroperitoneal and into the walls of the intestine). What fluid would you use to replace this and in what volume?
8. How necessary is admission to the ICU after operation? If a bed were not available, what would you do?
9. Consider the relative merits and disadvantages of regional and systemic analgesics after this operation.
10. What, overall, are the chances (percentage) of your patient surviving this operation to leave hospital?

Scenario 2

A 3-year-old boy presents to casualty with a history of acute onset of respiratory difficulty. He appears frightened but not overtly distressed. He has a respiratory rate of 40 breaths min^{-1}, a pronounced cough and biphasic stridor. He is not cyanosed breathing room air.

1. What is the differential diagnosis?
2. How could you establish the diagnosis?

A chest X-ray shows hyperinflation of the right lower zone.

3 What is the most likely diagnosis now?
4 What treatment is required?
5 Outline the anaesthetic management.

Scenario 3

You are called to A&E to assess a 24-year-old woman who has taken 50 co-proxamol tablets together with half a bottle of gin. She fitted intermittently in the ambulance and now has a Glasgow Coma Score (GCS) of 3:

1 What would you initially do for this patient?
2 Briefly discuss the immediate problems resulting from such an overdose.
3 What is the late complication of the overdose? How does it happen and how would you prevent it?

Scenario 4

A 20-year-old primigravida has requested epidural analgesia for her labour. She is extremely distressed despite pethidine, and her cervical dilatation is only 3 cm. While assessing the patient a question arises as to whether her membranes ruptured some time ago. In addition she has a temperature of 37.5 °C and a pulse rate of 100 bpm.

What do you do?

Scenario 5

The surgical senior house officer phones at 21:00 one night to book a 6-week-old boy in for an emergency pyloromyotomy. He has received fluid resuscitation for 3 hours, but is still a bit cool peripherally:

1 Describe the pathophysiology of pyloric stenosis.
2 Describe the biochemical abnormalities that characterize this condition.
3 What sort of fluid resuscitation would you use?
4 How would you anaesthetize this case?

Scenario 6

Scheduled for your ear, nose and throat list is a 70-year-old man with a laryngeal tumour for laryngectomy. He is a lifelong smoker who has rarely troubled his general practitioner until this illness. He occasionally uses a salbutamol inhaler; otherwise he is on no regular medication:

1   What are the potential anaesthetic problems this man may present?
2   What information would you like preoperatively?
3   How would you manage this case perioperatively?

Scenario 7

You are called to the ward at 23:00 to see a 10-year-old child who is 'crying out in pain'. He underwent a Nissen's fundoplication (painful upper midline abdominal wound) that morning and has a lumbar epidural infusion for postoperative analgesia. The child has severe cerebral palsy and mental retardation:

1   What difficulties might there be in assessing this child's pain?
2   What parameters might you use to assess his pain?
3   What additional information would be helpful?

Scenario 8

A 43-year-old male with chronic renal failure presents with an acute abdomen requiring a laparotomy:

1   How does chronic renal failure affect the different organ systems?
2   What are the important points in the preoperative assessment?
3   How should this patient be monitored perioperatively and what is a suitable anaesthetic technique?

Scenario 9

A 49-year-old insulin-dependent diabetic is to have a right below-knee amputation. His exercise is limited by his previous right forefoot amputation and he complains of dizziness on standing. He otherwise gives no medical history of note:

1   Which laboratory and bedside investigations should be performed?
2   Would a 6-hour fasting period ensure that he was adequately starved for theatre?
3   What factors would influence your preoperative insulin/glucose regimen?
4   Discuss the relative merits of general anaesthesia and central nerve blockade in a diabetic patient.

Scenario 10

A 24-year-old woman regurgitated and aspirated gastric contents on induction of general anaesthesia for Caesarean section. The baby was successfully delivered and the woman is transferred to ICU.

List 10 points that you consider important in her immediate management on ITU.

1 Although he seems relatively well, the risk of sudden rupture of his expanding aneurysm is very great. This is one of the few indications for emergency surgery (NCEPOD classification), i.e. within 1 hour. The others are 'urgent' (next opportunity, within 12 hours); scheduled (next opportunity), elective (when convenient). Many hospitals have a protocol for the management of acute aortic aneurysm and maintain equipment and drugs in readiness.

2 Justifiable operation – this is an otherwise fit man. Unless his ECG shows a recent silent infarction, his claim that he is fit is almost certainly true.

3 Monitoring preoperatively should be the minimum necessary to provide basic information. There should be no untoward delay. He should be taken directly into the operating theatre. Both arms should be placed on boards, abducted to a right angle. Monitoring at this stage should be confined to pulse oximetry. ECG and non-invasive automated blood pressure (set to 2-minute cycle). After induction, while the surgeon is making the initial incision, an arterial line and central venous pressure (CVP) can be introduced, together with two large i.v. cannulae. A surgical assistant should put in a urinary catheter.

4 Blood products will be needed, since stored blood will be given in quantity. A suggested minimum, to be requested before operation so that it is ready when the clamp is removed, is 2 units of fresh frozen plasma and 5 units of platelets. Warn the blood bank staff that more may be needed. Again, many hospitals have an agreed 'aneurysm protocol' for the provision of blood products.

5 When the surgeon cross-clamps the aorta (almost his first action after opening the abdomen), there is likely to be a sharp rise in arterial blood pressure, together with a large increase in systemic vascular resistance. Although controversial, most anaesthetists would start an infusion of sodium nitroprusside or glyceryl trinitrate at this point, titrating the dose to keep the blood pressure at the expected normal. During the cross-clamp period, give fluids to ensure a urine output of 60 ml per hour.

6 Cross-clamp release opens the aorta to flow and effectively reduces the systemic vascular resistance instantly. There is release of metabolites and vasodilatory substances into the circulation which may further influence both cardiac output and venous capacitance. Therefore before release of clamp:
   (i)   Preload the circulation so that the patient is fluid replete. Infuse colloid to raise the CVP to $10–15\ cmH_2O$.
   (ii) Have 4 units of blood ready.

   On release of the clamp:
   (i)   Infuse blood rapidly to keep the CVP to $10–15\ cmH_2O$.
   (ii) If necessary reduce or stop the vasodilator being used.
   (iii) Give 2 units of FFP and 5 units of platelets.
   (iv) Increase or commence an inotrope infusion to provide inotropic support if necessary.

7 The question of whether to use crystalloid or colloid to replace 'third space' losses is unresolved, which probably means that it does not matter which is used. Advocates of crystalloids claim increased urine output. Note that this

is a poor predictor of postoperative renal failure. Advocates of colloids claim improved postoperative respiratory function. A reasonable compromise is equal volumes of crystalloid and colloid, to keep the CVP about 10–15 cmH$_2$O and urine output above 60 ml per hour.

8 This patient will require close monitoring. Elective ventilation may be helpful to ensure maximum oxygenation and permit full analgesia. Renal and cardiovascular problems are likely. Optimal management in the first 24–48 hours is best conducted in an ICU or at least HDU environment. The benefits are:

- Cardiovascular system stability.
- Oxygenation.
- Early identification of bleeding.

9 Regional analgesia is relatively contraindicated because of possible coagulation problems after large volumes of stored blood. It may also be problematic if the patient is cardiovascularly unstable or has ongoing bleeding. Full parenteral analgesia is desirable to help avoid excessive sympathetic activity. Elective IPPV permits generous use of narcotics and good analgesia.

10 There are significant differences in outcome, depending on age, cardiac condition and the experience of the unit undertaking the procedure.

Further reading

Bayly PJ, Matthews JN, Dobson PM, Price ML, Thomas DG. In-hospital mortality from abdominal aortic surgery in Great Britain and Ireland: Vascular Anaesthesia Society audit. *Br J Surg* 2001; 88(5): 687–692

Pullman MD, Edwards ND. Current practice in the pre-operative assessment of patients for elective repair of abdominal aortic aneurysm: a survey of UK hospitals. *Anaesthesia* 1997; 52(4): 367–373

Volta CA, Verri M, Righini ER, Ragazzi R, Pavoni V, Alvisi R, Gritti G. Respiratory mechanics during and after anaesthesia for major vascular surgery. *Anaesthesia* 1999; 54(11): 1041–1047

Scenario 2

1 Differential diagnosis:

- Inhaled foreign body.
- Laryngotracheobronchitis (croup).
- Epiglottitis.
- Anaphylaxis with subglottic oedema.
- Asthma.
- Airway mass lesions: cyst, granuloma, lymphangioma.
- Inhalational burns.
- Hypertrophy of tonsils or adenoids.

2 Establishing the diagnosis:

- *History.* Acute onset favours foreign body inhalation or anaphylaxis. There may be a history of exposure to small objects (e.g. beads, coins) or (foods e.g. peanuts). There would normally be prodromal symptoms with croup or epiglottitis. Lesions in the airway would normally be known to the parents. Burns to the airway would follow exposure to fire or chemicals although this information may not always be forthcoming.

- *Examination.* Infectious causes would be expected to be associated with pyrexia. Children with epiglottitis classically appear toxic and drool saliva. An inhaled foreign body may be revealed by decreased breath sounds, hyper-resonance on percussion or wheezing.
- *Investigations.* The most useful investigation in this case is a chest X-ray. An inhaled foreign body may or not be visible but may be revealed by segmental hyperinflation, collapse or in long-standing cases such as pneumonia. In this case there is hyperinflation of the right lower zone.

3   As discussed above, this supports the diagnosis of inhaled foreign body, most probably in the right main bronchus.

4   The required treatment is bronchoscopy, usually rigid but sometimes flexible if the object is too distal to be reached by the rigid scope.

5   Anaesthetic management:

- Nurse the child with affected side dependent. Inhalational induction with $O_2 \pm N_2O$ and sevoflurane or halothane.
- Slowly progress until a deep plane of anaesthesia is obtained.
- Spray vocal cords with lignocaine.
- Once sufficiently 'deep', introduce bronchoscope.

Most authorities maintain that positive pressure ventilation should be avoided until the foreign body is removed. Anaesthesia can be maintained by attaching a T-piece to the bronchoscope side arm.

Humidified oxygen ± nebulized adrenaline may help to minimize postoperative subglottic oedema.

Further reading

Steen KH, Zimmermann T. Tracheobronchial aspiration of foreign bodies in children: a study of 94 cases. *Laryngoscope* 1990; 100: 525–530

Scenario 3

Paracetamol is predominantly metabolized in the liver by conjugation with either glucuronide or sulphate. A smaller proportion is metabolized by cytochrome P_{450} to a toxic reactive metabolite called *N*-acetyl-benzoquinonimine, which is then inactivated by conjugation with glutathione. In a large overdose, glutathione is depleted and the toxic metabolite reacts with hepatic proteins and binds covalently to liver cell membranes and hepatic necrosis results. Histologically it is predominantly centrilobular hepatic necrosis.

N-Acetylcysteine increases glutathione formation while thereby increasing conjugation. The risk of developing severe liver damage can be assessed from measuring the INR, seeing an elevated bilirubin, a raised creatinine, or elevated transaminases 24 hours or more following overdose. If this is the case, help from a specialized liver unit should be sought.

1 As with any unconscious patient, the ABC rules apply. A GCS of 3 indicates that the patient will be unable to protect her airway and so should be intubated, taking into account the presence of a full stomach.

2 Co-proxamol is a compound analgesic consisting of 32.5 mg dextropropoxyphene and 325 mg paracetamol per tablet. Dextropropoxyphene is an opioid structurally related to methadone. Taken in overdose, co-proxamol can result in death within 1 hour and as few as 15 tablets can be lethal. Toxicity is markedly enhanced by alcohol and death can occur within 15 minutes following combined ingestion. The initial features of overdose are related to dextropropoxyphene toxicity and consist of coma, respiratory depression, meiosis and cardiovascular collapse. In a large overdose, dextropropoxyphene is a negative inotrope and is associated with conduction abnormalities. Fitting is frequently seen.

   The patient must be swiftly resuscitated and then managed in an ICU setting. Intravenous naloxone (0.8–2 mg every 2–3 minutes, up to a maximum of 10 mg) should be given as an antagonist to the dextropropoxyphene. If this proves ineffective, then the diagnosis should be questioned.

3 Late complications are related to the paracetamol component of the tablet and early management should be directed towards preventing hepatotoxicity, which may not become apparent for 72–96 hours. Charcoal can be given orally or via a nasogastric tube to reduce drug absorption. The usefulness of gastric lavage is disputed. Guidance should be sought from the local poisons information centre. Patients at risk from hepatotoxicity can be identified from a plasma paracetamol level measured between 4 and 16 hours following the overdose. Levels measured before this may be misleading as they will not represent peak levels. By plotting on a graph the plasma paracetamol levels against time from ingestion, the need to treat with one of the antidotes can be determined. It should be noted that malnourished individuals or those on enzyme-inducing drugs can develop toxicity at much lower plasma paracetamol levels. Antidote treatment consists of either i.v. acetylcysteine or oral methionine. The antidotes are most effective if started within 10–12 hours of ingestion, although acetylcysteine is effective for up to 24 hours following overdose. If a potentially toxic dose of paracetamol has been taken, then treatment should be started prior to the plasma paracetamol level being known, although it can be stopped if the plasma concentration is subsequently found to be below the treatment level.

Further reading

Bessems JG, Vermeulen NP. Paracetamol (acetaminophen)-induced toxicity: molecular and biochemical mechanisms, analogues and protective approaches. *Crit Rev Toxicol* 2001; 31(1): 55–138

Gow PJ, Smallwood RA, Angus PW. Paracetamol overdose in a liver transplantation centre: an 8-year experience. *J Gastroenterol Hepatol* 1999; 14(8): 817–821

Scenario 4

This is a difficult problem! The major risk of performing an epidural on this patient is the seeding of infection into the CNS, resulting in either meningitis or an epidural abscess. Is it possible to decide if such a patient has a significant bacteraemia? The presence of tachycardia is of little use in this case because the link between temperature and bacteraemia is not reliable. Bacteraemia can occur in the absence of pyrexia and vice versa during labour. White blood cell count is raised in pregnancy and rises even further during labour, so most of our markers of systemic infection are not reliable.

How likely are infective sequelae following an epidural in this woman? Two studies reviewing both regional analgesia and anaesthesia in women with chorioamnionitis found no infective sequelae. If cases of meningitis and epidural abscess are reviewed, a clear link to a systemic infection is often not present, but failures in aseptic technique or repeated breaches of the CNS are frequently found.

Cases of haematological spread do occur but the incidence in our UK practice is unknown, but as we start auditing rare complications on a national basis this should change. The possible complications that could occur are very serious.

Regional anaesthesia is not the only form of analgesia available to this patient. Consideration should be given to other methods of analgesia and it should be ensured that they are used optimally.

Lastly, the patient needs to be fully informed of the risks should she still want to proceed to regional analgesia. But what exactly is the risk and what should you tell her? As in all such difficult cases, each one needs to be individually assessed and the risks and benefits considered.

Further reading

Swanson L, Madej TH. The febrile obstetric patient. In: Russell IF, Lyons G (eds). *Clinical Problems in Obstetric Anaesthesia*. Chapman & Hall, London, 1997

Scenario 5

1   Congenital pyloric stenosis is caused by gross thickening of the smooth muscle at the pylorus, resulting in gradual gastric outflow obstruction. It usually develops in the first 4–6 weeks of life and presents with vomiting that is characteristically described as projectile. Dehydration and weight loss ensue. The vomit may be blood stained as a result of gastritis and oesophagitis. It affects one in 500 births and has a male:female ratio of 4–6:1.

2   A hypochloraemic metabolic alkalosis with hypokalaemia is found. The vomiting results in the loss of H^+ and Cl^- as well as lesser amounts of Na^+ and K^+. The kidney responds by excreting alkaline urine. As K^+ is progressively

depleted, the kidney excretes H^+ rather than K^+ and so the urine becomes acidic, thus exacerbating the metabolic alkalosis. In severe cases, a lactic acidosis may be found. This is due to hypovolaemia and poor peripheral perfusion. Hypoglycaemia is a feature of such cases and this should be borne in mind throughout the anaesthetic management. The exact biochemical picture is influenced by the stage of the child presentation.

3   On admission, the urea and electrolytes and the acid–base status must be evaluated. The goal of resuscitation is to correct the dehydration, electrolyte disturbance and acid–base disturbance. A suitable fluid would be 5% dextrose and 0.45% NaCl with added K^+. Severely dehydrated cases may require colloid.

4   A skilled and experienced anaesthetist is essential and no surgery should be planned until a paediatric anaesthetist is available. If there is no one available the child must be transferred to a specialist paediatric surgical unit.

Clinically, the child has not received adequate resuscitation and surgery should not be carried out until this is so. Pyloromyotomy is not a surgical emergency and so the case can wait until a more suitable time. The urea and electrolytes and acid–base investigations must be reviewed, as surgery should not proceed until the child has been adequately rehydrated and the biochemical abnormalities corrected. This frequently takes 24–48 hours, but in severe cases this may take longer. The child's parents should be spoken to and a suitable history taken. Postoperative analgesia, including the possible use of suppositories, should be discussed. A nasogastric tube must be inserted preoperatively and the stomach must be aspirated prior to induction. As there is the potential for a full stomach, many would argue that a rapid-sequence induction is indicated. However, others would opt for a gaseous induction following careful stomach emptying. In the past, awake intubation was used.

Whichever method is chosen the child should be anaesthetised in a warm environment while oxygen saturation, blood pressure and ECG monitoring is in place. Paralysis and ventilation are used. At the end of the procedure, infiltration of the wound with local anaesthetic can be used, together with simple analgesic suppositories to keep the child comfortable. Opiates are not normally indicated. Children usually wake up quickly, although some are slow to start breathing. This may be the result of persisting cerebrospinal fluid alkalosis and intraoperative hyperventilation. Postoperative feeding regimes vary. Some units keep the children nil by mouth for up to 24 hours postoperatively. Intravenous fluids need to be prescribed during this period.

Further reading

MacDonald NJ, Fitzpatrick GJ, Moore KP, Wren WS, Keenan M. Anaesthesia for congenital hypertrophic pyloric stenosis. A review of 350 patients. *Br J Anaesth* 1987; 59: 672–677

Scenario 6

1   This man has been scheduled for major surgery. Despite his lack of past medical history the nature of this illness should raise a high index of suspicion to the presence of cardiorespiratory disease. Patients with laryngeal tumours

are often elderly and frail. They are very often smokers and are therefore likely to have cardiovascular and respiratory disease, which may have not been identified or investigated. The patient has presented with a laryngeal tumour so has a compromised airway. This may result in difficulty not only with intubation, but also with manual ventilation by face mask. In addition, the surgery planned involves the head and neck, giving limited access to the patient's airway and the need for perioperative tracheostomy formation. The surgery itself may be prolonged, with the potential for major blood loss, hypothermia, air embolism or pneumothorax.

2   Preoperatively a detailed history is required to ensure there are no symptoms of intercurrent illnesses which have not been identified. Subsequent investigations will need to be adjusted according to these findings. Minimum investigations would include full blood count, coagulation screen, urea and electrolytes, liver function tests, ECG and chest X-ray. Arterial blood gases and pulmonary function tests should be performed as he has a history of smoking and is at risk of postoperative respiratory complications; these investigations will help quantify any preoperative problem and give a useful baseline of his respiratory function. Any treatments which may improve the patient's preoperative state should be considered.

Next, attention needs to be paid to the airway problems. How did this man present? Specifically, the presence of stridor must be sought. The notes may give results of indirect laryngoscopy by the ear, nose and throat surgeons; he may even have had a biopsy under general anaesthesia where a previous chart may give a guide to ease of intubation and ventilation at that time. He may also have CT or MRI scans showing his airway. If the patient has received radiotherapy, this can result in scarring of the tissues, adding further difficulty to the airway management.

3   When planning the perioperative care of this man consideration of the following areas is required: the potential airway problem, the shared airway, access to the patient, potential blood loss, problems of prolonged surgery and his general medical state. Premedication with sedative drugs should be avoided if there is a risk of airway obstruction. Antisialogogues and bronchodilators may be indicated. Induction of anaesthesia is determined by the management of the airway. Depending upon the expected degree of difficulty, choices include awake fibre-optic intubation followed by intravenous induction or inhalation induction followed by intubation. Under inhalational anaesthesia it is possible to assess ease of ventilation and also to perform laryngoscopy to assess difficulty of intubation. Good venous access with appropriate extensions and fluid warmer are essential. Invasive monitoring allows close supervision of fluid balance, arterial blood gases and haematocrit. Other monitoring should include pulse oximetry, capnography, temperature and hourly urine output. Care must be taken when positioning the patient to protect pressure areas and the eyes. After positioning, it must be ensured that there is the ability to pull back the endotracheal tube during, and reattach the ventilation tubing after, tracheostomy formation. Steps should be taken against perioperative deep vein thrombosis by mechanical methods, such as calf compression or TED stockings and heels. Hypothermia should be avoided by the use of warming blankets and the warming of fluids

and inspired gases. Postoperatively this man requires care on an ICU or high-dependency unit where the staff are familiar with tracheostomies and he can be adequately monitored. He will require humidified oxygen therapy. Analgesia can be given via patient-controlled analgesia supplemented with NSAIDs if appropriate.

Scenario 7

1   The child may not understand the psychological tools and his/her behaviour may be misinterpreted by the behavioural scores. There is a genuine risk of either over- or under-treatment of this child's pain. Preoperative assessment is very useful to establish the child's normal behaviour and which, if any, pain tools are appropriate.

2   Physiological parameters such as heart rate, blood pressure, depth of respiration and oxygen saturation may be helpful.

3   Ask the child's guardian or parents. It is not uncommon to find that what appears to be distress is in fact the child's normal behaviour, compounded by anxiety.

Scenario 8

1   Initially there may be no indication of chronic renal failure, but as the disease progresses changes occur. There is polyuria and nocturia as the concentrating ability is lost and sodium and water are retained, causing volume overload. The ability to excrete potassium and hydrogen ions is lost, resulting in hyperkalaemia and acidosis. Abnormalities of calcium haemostasis and erythropoiesis may occur. The excretion of metabolic waste products such as urea is impaired. This is easy to measure, but it is not the urea as such that causes the problems we term 'uraemia' but the failure to excrete the thousands of other products of metabolism. In the cardiovascular system (CVS) there may be hypertension due to the increased circulating volume, which may precipitate congestive cardiac failure (CCF). Other factors implicated in CCF include the increased fluid load caused by the low colloid osmotic pressure of hypoalbuminaemia (in turn caused by the depression of enzyme systems resulting from increased toxic metabolite build-up), and the increased cardiac output necessary due to anaemia. Any pulmonary oedema can be worsened by calcium deposits in the myocardium and on the valves, which impairs contractility. Pericarditis, which is usually painful, may occur, as may pericardial effusions.

In the gastrointestinal system there is delayed gastric emptying due to autonomic neuropathy as well as an increased incidence of peptic ulcers, anorexia and vomiting. The skin becomes pigmented, the nails become brown and discoloured, and there is impaired wound-healing ability. Osteomalacia and osteosclerosis with bone pain may occur due to hyperparathyroidism, and muscle weakness may occur. In the CNS the effects of 'uraemia' may cause drowsiness, confusion and seizures: tiredness is due to anaemia. Peripheral and autonomic neuropathies may occur. In the endocrine system there is decreased erythropoietin synthesis and hyperparathyroidism. Platelet dysfunction occurs and bone marrow is suppressed. Both cellular and humoral defence mechanisms are impaired. Patients with chronic renal failure are also more likely to develop hypercholesterolaemia and gout.

2   Therefore, a full history and examination of the relevant organ systems should be performed. Features pertaining to fluid balance and time of last dialysis (in dialysis-dependent patients) should be ascertained. A history of exercise tolerance will indicate the severity of CVS disease and anaemia, but the patient should be specifically examined for signs of CCF and hypertension. The blood pressure should be taken and if possible the CVS assessed for autonomic neuropathy. It is important to ascertain fasting time for this patient as with any emergency patient. A history of epistaxis or bruising, or evidence of petechial haemorrhage, is an indication of platelet dysfunction A full blood count will provide information of anaemia and the number but not functional state of platelets. Serum electrolytes will show the degree of renal impairment (urea and creatinine), the potassium level and any disorder of sodium balance (usually hyponatraemia). Bicarbonate level may be reduced, indicating metabolic acidosis.

A particularly sick patient will warrant arterial blood gas analysis to assess acid–base status. An ECG is necessary as chronic renal failure patients have a higher incidence of myocardial infarction, hypertension and lipid abnormalities. Unless clinical examination indicates CCF a chest X-ray is not warranted.

3   In order to conduct a safe anaesthetic the patient should be well hydrated with an acceptable haemoglobin level. This is assessed with respect to any premorbid level that may be available and not by an accepted normal value. Care should be taken not to overload the patient while correcting any hypovolaemia. The potassium should ideally be less than 5 mmol l^{-1}. Any marked hyperkalaemia should be corrected with dextrose and insulin, salbutamol and/or bicarbonate infusion. An enquiry as to the sites of any dialysis shunts should be made so they can be avoided. Blood pressure should be monitored. This may be non-invasive if there is to be a prolonged procedure in a sick patient. An ECG is necessary to indicate any change in potassium levels which are manifest as T wave changes, as well as for rate and rhythm changes and for evidence of ischaemia. Pulse oximetry will give an early indicator of desaturation, which is important as the patient is already anaemic and any further reduction in oxygen delivery may be critical. Capnography helps to ensure that ventilation is adequate. The patient may already have a metabolic acidosis with a low bicarbonate, and any increase in carbon dioxide may cause a marked decrease in pH. Central line placement and other forms of invasive monitoring depend upon the severity of the patient's condition and fluid balance status. As soon as acceptable fluid balance is achieved, then one should proceed with general anaesthesia. In an emergency situation when the platelet function is unknown and fluid balance is likely to be difficult, a regional technique is not appropriate. With intravenous access secured, any stomach contents aspirated via a gastric tube and any invasive monitoring that is believed necessary in situ, a rapid-sequence induction should be performed. Less protein binding, a greater amount of non-ionized drug due to acidosis and greater permeability of the blood–brain barrier due to uraemia means that a less than usual induction dose of thiopentone is necessary.

Paralysis may be obtained by the use of suxamethonium if the serum potassium is normal, followed by atracurium. Alternatively, a high dose of atracurium (1 mg kg^{-1}) may be used if serum potassium is raised. Analgesic should be provided by short-acting opioid drugs such as fentanyl or alfentanil as the longer-acting drugs will accumulate. It is useful also to provide additional analgesia by wound infiltration with local anaesthetics. The volatile agent enflurane should be avoided if renal function is impaired. Atracurium should be reversed in the usual manner at the end of surgery. Postoperative care should ensure good analgesia, fluid balance and oxygenation.

Further reading

Cranshaw J, Holland D. Anaesthesia for patients with renal impairment. *Br J Hosp Med* 1996; 55: 171–175

Scenario 9

1 Bedside tests would include neurological examination, supine and erect blood pressures and Valsalva manoeuvre. Dense peripheral neuropathy, resting tachycardia, postural hypotension of > 30 mmHg and lack of heart variability on Valsalva manoeuvre are all indications of autonomic neuropathy. Laboratory tests include full blood count and random blood glucose, urea and electrolytes to assess dehydration and renal impairment. Electrocardiogram is helpful to assess past silent myocardial infarction, current ischaemia and ventricular strain (if associated with hypertension). A chest X-ray is not essential unless clinically indicated.

2 If he has an autonomic neuropathy, then complete gastric emptying preoperatively cannot by guaranteed and relevant precautions should be undertaken.

3 There are many GKI regimes in use and most hospitals have their own. A separate dextrose infusion and insulin sliding scale is useful for less well-controlled diabetics. A typical GKI regime may include 16 IU Actrapid and 10 mmol of potassium in 500 ml of 10% dextrose. However, the amount of insulin depends on the usual insulin requirements, current blood glucose and systemic illness of the patient. Potassium is adjusted according to serum potassium.

4 Specific advantages of regional techniques in diabetic patients include superior perioperative diabetic control, decreased risk of aspiration and superior blood gas exchange, since 25% of diabetics have impaired sensitivity to hypoxia or hypercarbia. Disadvantages include cardiovascular instability with central nerve blockade in the face of autonomic neuropathy. Most general anaesthetic agents cause mild hyperglycaemia which is of little clinical consequence.

Scenario 10

1 Oxygenate with 100% oxygen.
2 If particulate matter aspirated, perform bronchoscopy + lavage.

3 Positive end-expiratory pressure to control airway flooding.

4 Ventilation–pressure control/inverse ratio may be required.

5 Cardiovascular collapse may occur, requiring i.v. fluids/inotropes/PAOP.

6 Bronchodilator if wheeze present.

7 Steroids have not been shown to decrease mortality.

8 Prophylactic antibiotics are controversial; better to repeat frequent cultures.

9 Nasogastric tube to empty stomach, antacids, H_2 proton blockers.

10 IPPV, 10° head up to decrease risk of further aspiration.

Consider the following clinical scenarios as a presentation at a viva and review your answers to display judgement and prioritization. Remember that a display of knowledge without clinical interpretation is unlikely to impress the examiners, and that these answers are indicative only. You may disagree and have differing but equally acceptable answers.

Scenario 1

A 15-year-old boy presents at A&E with a 12-hour history of headache, fever and vomiting. On examination, his heart rate is 130 bpm, blood pressure 90/50 mmHg. He is confused and agitated. Capillary refill is 9 seconds.

1   What is your initial management?
2   What investigations should you do?

Scenario 2

A 26-year-old woman presents with intermittent vaginal bleeding at 36 weeks gestation. Her pulse rate is 90 bpm, blood pressure 110/70 mmHg. This is her second pregnancy, her first delivery being an emergency Caesarean section for failure to progress at term.

An ultrasound scan is performed, which shows a low-lying placenta that covers the internal os and the decision is taken to proceed to Caesarean section.

Discuss the anaesthetic management.

What are the chances of placenta accreta in this case?

Scenario 3

A young male has been resuscitated in casualty after sustaining major limb and abdominal trauma. He has been given large volumes of crystalloids and synthetic colloids in the absence of blood and blood product availability and he is now scheduled for emergency surgery.

1   Summarize the transfusion objectives prior to surgery.
2   What are the coagulation test parameters one would wish to achieve prior to surgery in the presence of active bleeding?
3   List the complications of massive transfusion.

Scenario 4

Allogenic blood is considered as a transplant from a voluntary donor to a recipient. The terminology used is the same as that for other tissue donation and the implications and consequences are similar.

1 What was allogenic blood formally known as?
2 What are the risks of transfusion?
3 What is thought to be one of the mediators of the blood storage defect?

Scenario 5

A 10-year-old boy with spina bifida is scheduled for multiple soft tissue releases to his right foot. Anaesthesia is induced and a laryngeal mask airway inserted. Some 10 minutes after the start of surgery the child's breathing becomes laboured and on examination it becomes apparent that he has severe bronchospasm and his upper torso is developing red blotches and wheals. He remains cardiovascularly stable.

1 What is happening?
2 Is the laryngeal mask airway contributing to this?
3 What is your immediate management?
4 Could this have been predicted?
5 What follow-up might be required?

Scenario 6

You are on call and late that evening the plastic surgeon refers a 14-year-old boy for toilet and suture of a laceration to his hand. When you go and see him it transpires that his mother is on holiday abroad and he is staying with his grandmother. He understands the nature of his injury and the proposed surgery and requests a general anaesthetic. His grandmother is with him and has signed the consent form.

1 Is this an emergency?
2 In Britain, what is the age of majority?
3 What is a 'mature minor' and who decides if this 14-year-old is a mature minor?
4 Who, therefore, has legal authority to consent to surgery and anaesthesia?
5 What would you do in this situation?

Scenario 7

You are asked to anaesthetize a 34-year-old woman for a cystoscopy. She suffered a traumatic spinal cord injury at T7, leaving her paraplegic 3 years previously. Despite this she is well, has no other past medical history, and has had previous uneventful general anaesthetics. You administer a general anaesthetic. Soon after the first incision she becomes markedly hypertensive (190/110 mmHg) and bradycardic (45 bpm). You notice her face is flushed and sweaty and her pupils are dilated.

1 What is the differential diagnosis?
2 What do you do next?
3 What stimuli can cause such a reaction in these patients?
4 What prophylaxis is available?

Scenario 8

A 6-year-old boy who had a tonsillectomy 6 hours ago is found to be restless and agitated on the post-surgical ward. He is tachycardic, clammy and nauseous.

1 What is the most likely cause of his condition?
2 What are the associated anaesthetic problems?
3 Outline your anaesthetic management?

Scenario 9

A 28-year-old man arrives in casualty at 23:00 after a road accident. He was allegedly knocked out at the scene but has been fully conscious since paramedics arrived. He has a compound fracture of his ankle, for which the orthopaedic surgeons are eager to take him to theatre. He now has a Glasgow Coma Scale score of 15 and has no other detectable injuries. Should the operation proceed tonight?

1 What are the main anaesthetic considerations?
2 Are any other investigations warranted?
3 What anaesthetic technique would you choose and why?

Scenario 10

A 38-year-old man presents for a day-case cystoscopy under general anaesthesia to investigate troublesome nocturia. He suffers from bronchiectasis and receives chest physiotherapy on a weekly basis. He frequently has infective exacerbations but feels well on the day of surgery. He also has asthma and takes regular inhaled steroids and salbutamol nebulizers four times a day. He has sensibly taken all his medication prior to arrival. He had a vasectomy as a day case 6 years previously under general anaesthesia without problems. His social circumstances are satisfactory.

Is this man suitable for day-case surgery? Give reasons for your decision.

Scenario 1

1　This boy is clearly severely shocked, with a very slow capillary refill despite only marginally low blood pressure. Therefore, initial management must be ABC with oxygen therapy, assessment of breathing and rapid i.v. or i.o. access. Blood cultures should be drawn when obtaining venous access if possible and antibiotics administered as soon as possible. While penicillin was conventionally used, high-dose cefotaxime is frequently used now. Resuscitation should begin with 20 ml kg^{-1} of colloid given as quickly as possible, and then reassess ABC. This history is very suggestive of septic shock with meningitis. Other signs such as neck stiffness and rash should be looked for as well as other causes of shock. A rash is highly suggestive of meningococcal infection. Early intubation is recommended as the situation may deteriorate rapidly and he is already confused and agitated. The patient should be admitted to an ICU or high-dependency unit at minimum.

2　A lumbar puncture will not change the initial management in a severely ill child and is relatively contraindicated if Glasgow Coma Scale score is < 13, in the presence of a coagulopathy or in the presence of any focal neurological sign. Similarly if this is meningococcal septicaemia then scanning is hazardous in a potentially unstable patient and will add very little. Blood cultures may be positive within hours.

3　The role of activated protein C could be discussed.

Further reading

Hodgetts TJ, Brett A, Castle NJ. The early management of meningococcal disease. *Accid Emerg Med* 1998; 15: 72–76

Riordan FA, Thomson AP. Recognition, treatment and complications of meningococcal disease. *Paediatr Drugs* 1999; 1: 263–282

Scenario 2

The potential problem here is catastrophic haemorrhage. This woman has been actively bleeding and has a placenta praevia and therefore runs a higher risk of substantial blood loss during Caesarean section (CS). Sixty-three per cent of all cases of placenta accreta present as placenta praevia. The combination of a previous CS and a placenta praevia means that she now has a 25% risk of a placenta accreta which may be associated with catastrophic haemorrhage. Although CS for placenta praevia may be carried out under regional blockade, the risk of placenta accreta with a previous CS, in a placenta already bleeding, would make a general anaesthetic safer in this context. This patient has a normal pulse rate and blood pressure for her gestation and has not lost an appreciable amount of blood. Sufficient time exists for adequate preparation and cross-matching of blood, which, where there is a risk of major obstetric haemorrhage, should include at least 4 units cross-matched, immediately available, two large-bore i.v. cannulae in place with blood warmers and a warming mattress. Both anaesthetist and surgeon should be of senior grade. Recovery facilities should be adequate for continuous monitoring of the patient as the risk of haemorrhage is still present postoperatively.

Further reading

Hunter T, Kleiman S. Anaesthesia for caesarean hysterectomy in a patient with a preoperative diagnosis of placenta percreta with invasion of the urinary bladder. *Can J Anaesth* 1996; 43: 24–51

Parekh N, Husaini SW, Russell IF. Caesarean section for placenta praevia: a retrospective study of anaesthetic management. *Br J Anaesth* 2000; 84: 725–730

Scenario 3

1 Summary of transfusion objectives:

- Transfuse to optimum filling pressures, mean arterial pressure and cardiac output.
- Optimize oxygen transport to the tissues.
- Avoid transfusion-induced hypothermia.
- Transfuse blood to maintain a haematocrit of 30–35%. Treat when the packed cell volume (PCV) is less than 28%. It is pointless giving blood when the PCV exceeds 40%.
- Give clotting factors to maintain prothrombin time (PT) and partial thromboplastin time (PTT) less than 1.8 times normal and fibrinogen levels greater than 1.5 g l^{-1}. These are for patients who are not actively bleeding or going to theatre.
- Dilutional thrombocytopenia should be treated with platelet concentrate to maintain platelets about 50×10^9 per litre.

These treatment objectives aim to maintain good tissue perfusion with adequate urine output in the face of threatened hypovolaemia and shock from blood loss. There is no need to transfuse blood initially as it has been shown that optimum rheology and viscosity occur at 30–35% in the fit, healthy patient. Blood product therapy in the form of fresh frozen plasma, cryoprecipitate and platelets may be necessary to achieve the coagulation parameters outlined.

2 Coagulation test parameters:

- Prothrombin time < 1.3 times control
- Partial thromboplastin time < 1.3 times control
- Thrombin time < 1.3 times control
- Fibrinogen > 100 mg/dl
- Activated coagulation time < 150 seconds

In the presence of active bleeding or the intention to proceed to surgery it is important to try and optimize the coagulation parameters further to avoid blood loss secondary to a coagulopathy. The reason for this tighter control is that the patient is likely to bleed as a consequence of surgery and the further volume expansion necessary will only make any dilutional coagulopathy worse. Prevention of blood loss due to poor coagulation is better than trying to treat the acquired defects of haemostasis once they have occurred.

3   The list shown is by no means complete but tries to include the major problems seen. The biochemical/acid–base derangements compounded by the citrate toxicity can cause severe impairment of myocardial performance even in previously fit patients and resultant hypotension and poor cardiac output is not uncommon. Treatment objectives should be aimed at prevention of these complications as soon as possible.

Acidosis	Micro-aggregates
Hypothermia	Hypocalcaemia
Dilutional coagulopathy	Hypophosphataemia
Altered O_2 delivery	Hypomagnesaemia
DIC	Hyperkalaemia (early)
Leucocyte sensitization	Hypokalaemia (late)
Complement activation	Citrate toxicity
Kinin activation	Impaired reticuloendothelial system
Vaso-occlusive disease	Transfusion reactions

Further reading

Harvey MP, Greenfield TP, Sugrue ME, Rosenfeld D. Massive blood transfusion in a tertiary referral hospital: clinical outcomes and haemostatic complications. *Med J Aust* 1995; 163(7): 356–359

Scenario 4

1   Donated blood was formally known as homologous blood, a homograft being the transplantation of tissue between members of the same species. The term autologous is the transfer of cells, tissue or organs back to the original donor.

2   The main risks of transfusion are:

- Complement-mediated ABO and Rh antigen antibody-induced haemolysis. This is the commonest cause of transfusion-related mortality but is extremely rare.
- Disease transmission, especially viral. AIDS and hepatitis C infections have caused recent concern. Solvent–detergent viral inactivation of fresh frozen plasma and cryoprecipitate has been successful in providing a safer form of these products but this technique is not possible with red blood cells as they are destroyed by the inactivation process. There is now unconfirmed concern about Creutzfeldt-Jakob disease.
- Immunosuppression is thought to be a cellular-mediated immunomodulation response to blood transfusion. Increased tolerance of transplanted organs, increased infection risks and early recurrence of neoplastic cells following tumour surgery have all been documented.

3   Recent evidence suggests that the presence of leucocytes in the stored blood may be one of the main factors in the development of the storage lesion. Filtration of blood to remove leucocytes has been shown to be beneficial, especially in the critically ill and immunosuppressed.

Further reading

Borghi B, Casati A. Incidence and risk factors for allogenic blood transfusion during major joint replacement using an integrated autotransfusion regimen: the Rizzoli Study Group on Orthopaedic Anaesthesia. *Eur J Anaesthesiol* 2000; 17(7): 411–417

Heiss MM, Fraunberger P, Delanoff C, Stets R, Allgayer H, Strohlein MA, Tarabichi A, Faist E, Jauch KW, Schildberg FW. Modulation of immune response by blood transfusion: evidence for a differential effect of allogenic and autologous blood in colorectal cancer surgery. *Shock* 1997; 8(6): 402–408

Scenario 5

1 This child is having an allergic reaction with the release of substances such as histamine, resulting in bronchospasm and urticaria. While he has been exposed to a number of potentially allergenic agents during his anaesthetic, a potential culprit in this situation is latex. Children with spina bifida who self-catheterize are at high risk of developing anaphylactic reactions to latex. The clinical severity will vary and may be life-threatening.

2 Laryngeal mask airways are not made from latex and are safe. However, in this situation serious consideration should be given to exchanging for an endotracheal tube in case of oedema causing upper airway obstruction.

3 Resuscitation should follow the priorities of 'airway, breathing, circulation'. Intravenous β_2-agonists may be sufficient to relieve simple bronchospasm, but if the reaction is more severe then management should include prompt treatment with intravenous adrenaline and volume replacement following the Association of Anaesthetists guidelines for the management of major anaphylaxis. Remove and/or discontinue all likely allergens and terminate surgery.

4 In addition to a history of self-catheterization, evidence of marked sensitivity to everyday items containing rubber, such as balloons or swimming caps, may be found, increasing the chance of a reaction in theatre.

4 It is necessary to establish that an anaphylactic reaction has taken place and then investigate the possible causative agents. At the time of the reaction, serum should be taken to look for an elevated tryptase, which will confirm an anaphylactic reaction, i.e. mast cell degranulation. A referral to an appropriate local specialist should be made to arrange either skin prick testing or radio-allergo-absorbent testing for likely triggering agents.

Further reading

Kemp SF, Lockey RF, Wolf BL, Lieberman P. Anaphylaxis. A review of 266 cases. *Arch Intern Med* 1995; 155(16): 1749–1754

Thacker MA, Davis FM. Subsequent general anaesthesia in patients with a history of previous anaphylactoid/anaphylactic reaction to muscle relaxant. *Anaesth Intensive Care* 1999; 27(2): 190–193

Scenario 6

1   No. There is a degree of urgency, but this is not an emergency.

2   In Britain the age of majority is 18. However, the Family Reform Act of 1969 states that once a person reaches the age of 16 they are able to consent to treatment. The reverse is not necessarily true and this age group may not be able to refuse treatment in some circumstances.

3   A child who is deemed able to completely understand the nature and consequences of a given procedure and alternative choices is said to be a mature minor or 'Gillick competent'. A child may be mature enough to consent to an adenoidectomy, but the same child may not be able to consent to chemotherapy because of its more serious nature. The decision whether a child is mature enough to give consent seems to rest with the doctor.

4   In general, parents have the authority to make decisions on behalf of their legally incompetent children. But in this case this child may be judged competent and, therefore, able to give consent on his own behalf. Consent given by grandparent is invalid.

5   Notwithstanding the child's maturity, prudence may suggest that this non-emergency surgery be deferred for a period while reasonable efforts are made to contact his mother abroad.

Scenario 7

1   The two most likely diagnoses are:

- Inadequate depth of anaesthesia.
- Autonomic hyperreflexia.

Other more unlikely diagnoses that would fit this pattern include raised intracranial pressure and possibly myocardial ischaemia.

2   The initial treatment for the first two diagnoses is the same:

- Withdraw the surgical stimulus.
- Deepen the plane of anaesthesia.

If the clinical picture settles then inadequate anaesthesia alone can be assumed and the operation can continue under the deeper anaesthetic.

If the situation fails to resolve then autonomic hyperreflexia is the likely cause and prompt treatment is required.

- Call for help.
- Pharmacological intervention to lower blood pressure.
    - Sodium nitroprusside.
    - Calcium channel blockers.
    - Heart rate should increase as blood pressure returns to normal, but persistent bradycardia can be treated with anticholinergics.
    - Invasive arterial monitoring is helpful to accurately monitor treatment effectiveness.
    - Postoperative monitoring is essential and should probably take place on ICU/high-dependency unit.

3 Virtually any stimulus below the level of the spinal cord lesion may provoke autonomic hyperreflexia in these patients. In order of frequency they include:

- Genitourinary, especially bladder distension.
- Gastrointestinal, e.g. sigmoidoscopy.
- Others – many and varied but includes temperature extremes and tight clothing.

4 Prophylactic measures include:

- Pretreatment with calcium channel blockers.
- Ensuring adequate depth of anaesthesia before surgery starts.
- Regional anaesthesia, especially subarachnoid, is effective in blocking the surgical stimulus but may be difficult to perform in these patients.

Further reading

Ahmed AB, Bogod DG. Anaesthetic management of a quadriplegic patient with severe respiratory insufficiency undergoing caesarean section. *Anaesthesia* 1996; 51(11): 1043–1045

Amzallag M. Autonomic hyperreflexia. Int *Anesthesiol Clin* 1993; 31(1): 87–102

Habibi A, Schmeising C, Gerancher JC. Interscalene regional anesthesia in the prevention of autonomic hyperreflexia in a quadriplegic patient undergoing shoulder surgery. *Anesth Analg* 1999; 88(1): 98–99

Scenario 8

1 The diagnosis is most likely to be primary post-tonsillectomy bleed. The general appearances are consistent with bleeding, and the restlessness and tachycardia would suggest hypovolaemia.

2 The anaesthetic problems are hypovolaemia, coupled with a full stomach containing the 'hidden' blood loss. Clot or active bleeding in the pharynx may make intubation difficult. The residual effects of the original anaesthetic agents need to be considered.

3 General anaesthesia is required to allow surgical control of the haemorrhage. First, good intravenous access needs to be established. Intravascular volume replacement is necessary prior to anaesthesia. A rapid-sequence induction is employed for induction of anaesthesia by most anaesthetists. The dose of induction agent should be reduced and suction equipment readily available and functioning. Following intubation, the stomach should be evacuated of blood with an orogastric tube. Care should be taken to avoid further trauma on insertion. The child should be extubated awake in the lateral position to minimize the risk of airway obstruction.

Further reading

Steward DJ. *The Manual of Pediatric Anesthesia. Hospital for Sick Children.* Toronto, Canada, 1990: 100–102

1 Ideally any compound fracture should be debrided as soon as possible, usually taken to mean within 6 hours of presentation. Therefore, as long as there are no other injuries requiring more urgent treatment (including head injury – see below), then the operation should proceed as planned.

2 The main concern is whether or not a significant head injury has been sustained. He was reputedly unconscious so a head injury did occur and as this is suspected then the following questions need to be answered:

- Are further investigations needed?
- Does treatment for any intracranial pathology take precedence over the compound fracture?
- Assuming the answers to the above are negative, would an anaesthetic for ankle debridement compromise further monitoring/assessment of the patient's neurological status?

As there has been loss of consciousness a skull X-ray is indicated. Whether this shows a fracture or is inconclusive, a CT of the head should be performed. This will be determined by clinical circumstance and would be the safest option if an anaesthetic is considered essential. The positive yield is likely to be very low.

3 The choice of anaesthetic technique is from:

- *General anaesthetic.* The advantages are that it has a very low failure (i.e. awareness) rate and it is not limited by duration of operation. The disadvantages include the regurgitation risk, interference with monitoring of neurological status, raised intracranial pressure if hypercarbia and high concentrations of volatile used.
- *Subarachnoid block.* The advantage is that there is no interference with consciousness level. The disadvantages are the potential for 'coning' if intracranial pressure is raised and that the duration of block is limited.
- *Extradural anaesthesia.* The advantage is the same as for subarachnoid, but a continuous catheter technique can be used to prolong anaesthesia for as long as required. The disadvantage is that an accidental dural puncture may occur.
- *Combined femoral/sciatic block.* This is, theoretically, probably the ideal technique, as anaesthesia is limited to the affected limb only. The real disadvantages are that the failure rate is relatively high, the technique is not as familiar to many anaesthetists, and large doses of local anaesthetic are required with potential for toxicity, which may cloud the clinical picture. In practice it is therefore not the ideal technique.

This man has respiratory disease that significantly affects his daily life. He is therefore unsuitable to have a general anaesthetic on a day-case basis. The risk of perioperative respiratory complications is high both from anaesthesia-related atelectasis with subsequent respiratory difficulty and from precipitation of an acute asthma attack. The fact that he has had a general anaesthetic on a day-case basis previously is encouraging, but should not be the sole determinant for selection.

A planned overnight admission with chest physiotherapy pre and post surgery would be more suitable should general anaesthesia be necessary.

Other possibilities: one must also remember that an alternative procedure under local anaesthesia may be possible; a flexible cystoscopy would be the preferable diagnostic procedure in this case. Minimizing the time spent in hospital also reduces the risk of this man becoming colonized with a resistant organism or developing a hospital-acquired chest infection.

Further reading

Cammu G, Smith I. Day surgery, including the preoperative assessment of the patient: a UK experience by a Belgian anaesthetist. *Acta Anaesthesiol Belg* 2000; 51(3): 173–185

Consider the following clinical scenarios as a presentation at a viva and review your answers to display judgement and prioritization. Remember that a display of knowledge without clinical interpretation is unlikely to impress the examiners, and that these answers are indicative only. You may disagree and have differing but equally acceptable answers.

Scenario 1

A 25-year-old primigravida at 32 weeks' gestation presents to the Accident and Emergency Department complaining of headache. Soon after arrival she has a generalized seizure lasting 3 minutes. She has had no antenatal care and is accompanied by a neighbour who believes her to be normally fit and well.

1　What is the differential diagnosis?
2　What investigations are required immediately?
3　Outline your plan of treatment up to and including delivery.
4　What complications could be expected after delivery?

Scenario 2

A 26-year-old man presents for examination and repair of a penetrating eye injury, sustained during an alleged assault. His injury was sustained approximately 2 hours prior to presentation. He has also sustained other facial injuries including an undisplaced fracture of the mandibular ramus.

1　Outline the main points of the preoperative assessment of this patient.
2　What factors will influence the timing of the procedure?
3　What are the available options for the induction of anaesthesia? Briefly outline their advantages and disadvantages.

Scenario 3

A 55-year-old man is listed for a total knee replacement. He is a little overweight and gives a history of a hiatus hernia diagnosed at endoscopy. His past medical history is otherwise unremarkable, but he is found to be hypertensive, with a blood pressure of 180/110 mmHg. An ECG and blood tests are normal. After observation overnight his blood pressure settles to 150/100 mmHg. A general anaesthetic with nerve blocks is planned and a benzodiazepine prescribed before theatre.

1　Are any other assessments or investigations indicated? Would you plan a different anaesthetic?

With routine monitoring in place, a rapid-sequence induction with fentanyl, thiopentone and suxamethonium is undertaken. Direct laryngoscopy gives a good view and intubation is accomplished without delay. The patient immediately becomes markedly tachycardic and sweaty, developing red flushing around his face and neck.

2　What are the most likely causes of this reaction?

On checking, his blood pressure is 240/120 mmHg and he begins to have multiple ventricular ectopics. His chest is clear.

3　What causes must be considered?
4　How would you manage this?

Scenario 4

A 35-year-old woman presents for total abdominal hysterectomy. She is noted to have ptosis, frontal balding, intellectual impairment and an inability to relax muscles after contraction.

1　What underlying inherited disease is present?
2　Describe the pathophysiology, symptoms and signs of the disease.
3　How would you anaesthetize this patient?

Scenario 5

An otherwise fit 54-year-old man is listed for an L3–L4 discectomy. He is induced with fentanyl, propofol and atracurium and is intubated. Anaesthesia is maintained with nitrous oxide, oxygen and isoflurane with an inspired oxygen concentration of 35%. The patient is transferred to the operating table and safely place in the prone position. He is monitored with ECG, NIBP, SpO2, ETCO$_2$, FiO$_2$, agent monitor and PNS. Initial dissection and identification of the correct lumbar level with X-ray is uneventful. While removing disc material, the patient becomes increasingly hypotensive and tachycardic. When you look at the patient he has a thin thready pulse, air entry to both lung fields and heart sounds can be heard. There is no rash or oedema. The pulse oximeter reads 97%, the complexes on the ECG are unchanged and airway pressures are stable. There is no air in the intravenous lines. When you mention this to the surgeon he says there was a brief welling of blood into the surgical field a little earlier.

1　In this situation what could be the possible causes of a sudden drop in blood pressure?
2　Which important diagnosis must be considered and treated if appropriate?
3　How common is this?
4　What mortality does it carry?
5　What is your plan of action now?

Scenario 6

You are asked to site an epidural for analgesia in a primigravida at 38 weeks' gestation who is in the early stages of labour. She has no coexisting disease, has no contraindications to epidural analgesia and has received Entonox only for analgesia. After explanation of the technique she gives verbal consent for you to proceed. You being insertion with a 16-gauge Tuohy needle at the L3–L4 interspace. However, she is becoming increasingly distressed by the contraction pains and moves suddenly as a contraction starts. At this moment you notice a free flow of clear fluid from the proximal end of the Tuohy needle.

1 Outline your immediate management of the situation, and your plan of management for the remainder of her labour.
2 What problem may this patient develop in the early puerperium? How likely is this to occur? What therapeutic options are available to you?
3 Are there any analgesic strategies available which may have prevented this situation occurring?

Scenario 7

A 40-year-old male patient is booked as an urgent case for tracheostomy and percutaneous endoscopic gastrostomy (PEG). The patient has a large tumour infiltrating most of the tongue, oropharynx and extending into the neck. At the time of diagnosis the patient refused surgery. Unfortunately, the tumour did not respond to radiotherapy. Now, he can just swallow saliva and liquid diet but cannot swallow solids.

1 Describe your anaesthetic management of this patient.
2 List the complications of tracheostomy.

Scenario 8

A 40-year-old woman with a history of myasthenia gravis presents to casualty with a 2-day history of increasing head and neck weakness and difficulty breathing. Over the last 2 hours she had become acutely short of breath, with associated drowsiness. She had given birth by normal vaginal delivery 1 week earlier. She underwent thymectomy for a myasthenic crisis 10 years ago and she took an overdose of pyridostigmine 4 years ago. Her current medications are pyridostigmine, prednisolone and azathioprine.

1 What factors may have contributed to the muscle weakness?
2 Describe your initial management.
3 What are the problems involved in anaesthetising a patient with myasthenia gravis?

Scenario 9

You are in the obstetric theatre caring for a woman having a routine Caesarean section under epidural anaesthesia. The baby is delivered and has an immediate Apgar score of 7. The midwife suddenly notices that the baby goes blue and apnoeic when its mouth is closed. There is no paediatrician present because of an emergency in the next theatre. The midwife asks for your help and advice.

1   What is the likely cause?
2   What is the immediate treatment?
3   Describe the condition embryologically.
4   What preoperative investigations are necessary?
5   What is the surgical treatment?
6   Describe a safe anaesthetic technique.

Scenario 10

A 40-year-old man is scheduled on your list for uvulopharyngopalatoplasty (UPPP). He was found to be mildly hypertensive on admission (170/110 mmHg), and his haemoglobin is raised at 18 g dl^{-1}. His body mass index (BMI) is 40. When you see him preoperatively you find him asleep. He is making severe paradoxical attempts to breathe, and gasps into wakefulness as you arrive at his bed. While you question him you notice that he is still struggling to stay awake.

1   What is the likeliest diagnosis?
2   What is the calculation for the BMI?
3   What are the anaesthetic problems of patients with this problem?
4   What would you do tonight?
5   What formal investigations are necessary?
6   What is the appropriate treatment of this man?

1 Convulsions occurring in the later stages of pregnancy should be regarded as eclampsia unless proven otherwise. However, the differential diagnosis would include:

- Epilepsy.
- Intracranial haemorrhage or infarction.
- Intracranial space-occupying lesion.
- Meningitis or encephalitis.
- Hypoglycaemia.
- Systemic lupus erythematosis.

2 Initial investigations that would help to establish the diagnosis include:

- Arterial blood pressure. Likely to be very high (systolic greater than 160 mmHg or diastolic greater than 110 mmHg) in eclampsia.
- Urinalysis. Marked proteinuria would also support the diagnosis of eclampsia.
- Blood glucose measurement. To exclude hypoglycaemia as a cause or result of the seizure.
- CT scan. If none of the above investigations reveal any abnormality, or focal signs are present, a CT scan may be indicated to look for intracranial pathology.

Other immediate investigations in suspected eclampsia:
- Full blood count and clotting studies. To rule out thrombocytopenia, haemolysis or a disseminated intravascular coagulopathy.
- Serum electrolytes. May show an elevated creatinine and will exclude electrolyte disturbance as a cause of the seizure.

Other investigations will be required, e.g. liver function tests, but are not essential (or often available) immediately.

3 Management can be considered under the following headings:

- *Immediate management*. The patient should be placed in the left lateral position and the airway secured, by intubation if necessary. Supplemental oxygen should be administered and intravenous access established. The goal of subsequent management is to limit maternal and fetal morbidity pending delivery of the fetus, the only definitive treatment for eclampsia.
- *Treatment and prophylaxis of seizures*
  Seizures should be controlled and further seizures prevented with anticonvulsants. The first-line drug in this situation is intravenous magnesium sulphate. If repeated seizures occur despite magnesium, options include diazepam or thiopentone (increments of 50 mg). In such situations intubation is likely to be required.
- *Treatment of hypertension*. Reduction of severe hypertension (greater than 160/100 mmHg or mean greater than 125 mmHg) is essential to decrease the risk of cerebrovascular accident. This may be achieved with either hydralazine (up to 20 mg in 5 mg increments over 20 minutes) or labetolol (up to a maximum dose of 300 mg). Consideration should be made to direct intra-arterial measurement of blood pressure to guide therapy.

- *Fluid therapy*. Close monitoring of fluid therapy and urine output is mandatory. Preloading the circulation with up to 500 ml of colloid solution should be considered before vasodilation. Thereafter, fluid therapy should be limited to maintenance crystalloid.
- *Investigations*. Frequent monitoring of haemoglobin, platelet count, transaminases, urea and creatinine should be performed. Oxygen saturation should be monitored continuously.
- *Delivery*. This is the definitive treatment but should not be considered until the mother is stable. A Caesarean section under general anaesthesia is indicated in this patient. A rapid-sequence induction should be performed with the usual precautions for an obstetric patient. However, preparations should be made for a difficult intubation owing to laryngeal oedema. Consideration should be given to attenuating the pressor response to intubation with, for example, a short-acting opioid such as alfentanil. Patients who have received magnesium will need close monitoring of neuromuscular function as the action of non-depolarizing muscle relaxants may be potentiated. The patient should be transferred to an intensive therapy unit postoperatively.

4 Complications of hypertensive disorders of pregnancy include:

- Stroke.
- Haemolysis, elevated liver enzymes and low platelets.
- Disseminated intravascular coagulopathy.
- Renal failure.
- Pulmonary oedema.
- Aspiration of gastric contents.
- Acute respiratory distress syndrome.

Further reading

Roberts JM, Cooper DW. Pathogenesis and genetics of pre-eclampsia. *Lancet* 2001; 357(9249): 53–56

Taner CE, Hakverdi AU, Aban M, Erden AC, Ozelbaykal U. Prevalence, management and outcome in eclampsia. *Int J Gynaecol Obstet* 1996; 53(1): 11–15

Scenario 2

1 As with any patient presenting for surgery a full history and physical examination are mandatory. Supplementary investigations may be required. Particular points of note in the history include:

- The nature of the assault.
- The presence of significant head injury, i.e. loss of consciousness, neurological symptoms, etc.
- Other significant injuries, including dental trauma.
- The duration of preoperative fasting and the timing of the last oral intake in relation to the injury. An estimate of drug intake, alcohol or other substances is also important at this stage.
- Has a significant amount of blood been swallowed?

The physical examination should include a full neurological examination and a thorough airway examination to predict ease of intubation. Particular attention should be paid to mouth opening as he has sustained a mandibular fracture at the same time. The two main anaesthetic factors that may delay surgery are a coexisting head injury and a potentially full stomach.

2 Any decision regarding the timing of the procedure should be taken in consultation with the ophthalmologist and the oral surgeon, if consideration is being given to fixing the mandibular fracture at the same time. Most penetrating eye injuries can be delayed if necessary and should be delayed to allow for neurological evaluation or for the stomach to empty. There is no urgency to fix the mandible.

3 The principal aims of the anaesthetic technique in this situation are protection of the airway with avoidance of marked increases in intraocular pressure (IOP), which could result in extrusion of ocular contents. As with most trauma patients, this patient must be considered to have a full stomach. Although, as discussed earlier, surgery may be delayed for a short time, emptying of the stomach cannot be guaranteed. For this reason, together with the need to control carbon dioxide tension and thus IOP, tracheal intubation is required.

No attempt should be made preoperatively to empty the stomach with a nasogastric or orogastric tube as the retching it is likely to provoke will raise IOP significantly. Unless there is a good history of pre-injury starvation a rapid-sequence or modified rapid-sequence induction will be required. Pre-oxygenation should be performed with care to avoid pressure on the affected eye from the face mask and pain at, or distraction of, the fracture site. With the exception of ketamine, all the induction agents in common use lower IOP and may be used. The main controversy surrounding this procedure involves the choice of muscle relaxant used to facilitate intubation. Suxamethonium is an essential component of rapid-sequence induction, but it causes a rise in IOP. Despite this theoretical disadvantage, evidence that it leads to extrusion of eye contents is lacking. However, airway protection must take precedence, and where intubation may prove difficult, as in this case, it is a wise precaution to use suxamethonium.

Many modifications of this technique and alternatives to it have been described in an attempt to avoid this rise in IOP. These are outlined below:

Priming

Pretreatment with small subparalytic doses of suxamethonium before the full intubating dose has been tried but with little success. Pretreatment with small doses of non-depolarizing relaxants have shown variable limitations to suxamethonium-induced increases in IOP. Some patients show unexpected sensitivity to these doses, however, which makes this technique inappropriate in a patient in whom it may be difficult to maintain or secure an airway. Priming with other agents, e.g. intravenous diazepam, lignocaine, opioids, β-blockers and acetazolamide, has been tried but is of questionable benefit.

Alternatives to suxamethonium

A non-depolarizing relaxant could be used as part of a modified rapid-sequence induction. Priming with subparalytic doses of relaxant may decrease the onset time but has the disadvantages outlined above. Larger than normal doses of rocuronium reliably produce sufficient muscle relaxation for intubation within 60 seconds. However, the duration of action is also prolonged and this technique is therefore inappropriate if difficulty in airway control is anticipated.

Obtunding the pressor response to laryngoscopy and intubation

Laryngoscopy and intubation regardless of the relaxant used cause an increase in IOP, which may be attenuated with lignocaine (intravenously or by nebulizers), nifedipine, β-blockers, opioids or supplemental doses of induction agent.

The suspected difficult airway

Should mouth opening be severely limited, or there are other features which suggest difficulty in intubation or airway compromise, then an awake fibre-optic or gas induction should be considered. These, however, are likely to result in coughing or straining with resultant increases in IOP. As previously stated, however, control of the airway must take precedence, if necessary at the expense of intraocular contents.

Scenario 3

1   This man's initial hypertension was attributed to his weight and his understandable anxiety on admission to hospital for an operation. It subsequently settled to a more reasonable level and was accompanied by normal blood tests and ECG. It may have been worth enquiring whether his GP had seen him recently and taken his blood pressure, for comparison. An alternative anaesthetic technique would have been to offer a spinal anaesthetic or combined spinal epidural, particularly in view of his hiatus hernia.

2   Inadequate anaesthesia or an adverse reaction possibly from suxamethonium would immediately spring to mind as the cause of this reaction. Malignant hyperthermia is unlikely but may produce this picture initially.

3   In a hypertensive who is not on treatment it could be an exaggerated hypertensive response but this would be unusual. The possibility of an undiagnosed phaeochromocytoma manifesting itself with a surge of catecholamines following the stimulation of intubation must be considered. This may be linked to conditions such as neurofibromatosis. In addition, carcinoid tumours can on occasion cause hypertension rather than hypotension, along with flushing and bronchospasm.

4   The diagnosis will not be clear at this stage, but its serious nature and the need for decisive action will be. The operation is entirely elective in nature and should be postponed. Supportive treatment is given. 100% oxygen

should be administered and a plan made to wake the patient as soon as the suxamethonium has worn off. It may be wise to substitute an intravenous agent such as propofol for volatile agents to avoid further possible triggering of malignant hyperthermia. Good intravenous access should be secured and intravenous fluids commenced at an appropriate rate. Arterial blood gases would be extremely helpful in making a diagnosis and guiding management. Specific therapy then depends upon subsequent events. In this case the patient's blood pressure remained very high. His blood gases were essentially normal with no hyperkalaemia or acidosis. He remained apyrexial. A provisional diagnosis of a phaeochromocytoma was made and he was initially treated with phentolamine before being transferred to the intensive care unit for further treatment and observation. Alternative agents could have been glycerol trinitrate or sodium nitroprusside and with sustained blood pressure and tachycardia but without failure a β-blocker may have been useful. The diagnosis was later confirmed by finding increased levels of vanillylmandelic acid in a urine sample.

Further reading

Beatty OL, Russell CF, Kennedy L, Hadden DR, Kennedy TL, Atkinson AB. Phaeochromocytoma in Northern Ireland: a 21 year review. *Eur J Surg* 1996; 162(9): 695–702

Hirsch NP, Murphy A, Radcliffe JJ. Neurofibromatosis: clinical presentations and anaesthetic implications. *Br J Anaesth* 2001; 86(4): 555–564

Holdcroft A. Hormones and the gut. *Br J Anaesth* 2000; 85(1): 58–68

Kinney MA, Warner ME, Nagorney DM, Rubin J, Schroeder DR, Maxson PM, Warner MA. Perianaesthetic risks and outcomes of abdominal surgery for metastatic carcinoid tumours. *Br J Anaesth* 2001; 87(3): 447–452

Scenario 4

1 The diagnosis is dystrophia myotonica.
2 This is an autosomal dominant disease with variable penetrance. An abnormality of calcium metabolism in skeletal, smooth and cardiac muscle results in continued contraction after stimulation. There is a mutation on chromosome 19 in 99% of cases. Males and females are equally affected. The usual onset is between 15 and 40 years. It is a systemic disease, with progressively more severe symptoms and signs with succeeding generations ('anticipation'). There are characteristic histological changes within muscle fibres of long chains of central nuclei, eventually progressing to necrosis and fibrosis. Myotonia results in an inability to relax muscles after voluntary use or in response to mechanical stimulation. Cold, exercise, hyperkalaemia and shivering may precipitate myotonia. There is weakness and atrophy of facial muscles, sternocleidomastoid, the shoulder girdle and quadriceps. Muscle reflexes are lost. An abnormal facies is present with frontal balding, ptosis, cataracts, a smooth forehead and a lateral smile. Testicular or ovarian atrophy is associated with impotence and sterility. Other associated

disorders include mental deformity, glucose intolerance, cholelithiasis, delayed gastric emptying, pharyngeal dystrophy, cardiomyopathy, conduction disorders, cardiac failure and respiratory muscle weakness. Electromyography shows spontaneous myotonic discharges. Phenytoin, procainamide or quinine may help the myotonia. Genetic counselling is required. Death usually occurs in the sixth decade owing to cardiac or respiratory failure.

3 A careful preoperative assessment is made for cardiac involvement, pulmonary infection and respiratory failure. Preoperative investigations include U & Es, ECG and pulmonary function tests. Premedication is avoided as there is increased sensitivity to all depressant drugs. Invasive cardiovascular monitoring (including pulmonary artery catheter) may be indicated. Temperature is monitored. Intravenous induction may be used with the smallest possible dose of induction agent. Thiopentone is known to be safe, although there may be increased sensitivity with prolonged apnoea. A low dose of propofol is reported to be safe. Gas induction may be used, but respiratory weakness may be a problem and conduction disorders may progress to more extensive heart block. All muscle relaxants are avoided if possible. Suxamethonium may induce severe myotonia, which may result in complete inability to intubate or ventilate. There is a variable response to non-depolarizing muscle relaxants, with either a normal response, increased sensitivity or myotonia. Atracurium may be the agent of choice, but monitoring of neuromuscular function is essential. Other factors which trigger myotonia (shivering, halothane, hyperkalaemia) are avoided. There is increased sensitivity to opioids and volatile agents. Regional anaesthesia cannot guarantee prevention of myotonia but may offer advantages by avoiding depressant opioids for perioperative analgesia. Neostigmine may precipitate myotonia – ventilation should continue until spontaneous recovery of neuromuscular function. Injection of local anaesthetic into the muscle itself may modify myotonia. Postoperatively, intensive care may be required for ventilation for slow recovery of consciousness, prolonged neuromuscular blockade or cardiovascular instability. Early feeding is avoided since impaired swallowing and delayed gastric emptying result in a high incidence of aspiration.

Further reading

Imison AR. Anaesthesia and myotonia – an Australian experience. *Anaesth Intensive Care* 2001; 29(1): 34–37

Russell SH, Hirsch NP. Anaesthesia and myotonia. *Br J Anaesth* 1994; 72(2): 210–216

1 The causes of this fall in blood pressure include:

- Anaphylaxis.
- Hypovolaemia.

- Air embolism.
- Pulmonary embolism.
- Cardiac tamponade.
- Pneumothorax.
- Cardiac event.

2   Which important diagnosis must be considered and treated if appropriate? This patient is showing signs of hypovolaemia but not obviously losing blood. If an epidural vein had been torn the blood loss is usually overt. However, covert and catastrophic bleeding may occur into the retroperitoneal space if the aorta or inferior vena cava is 'nibbled' accidentally during discectomy owing to their close association with the spine and, therefore, the discs. A high index of suspicion is needed because only rapid action will save the patient.

3   This problem is estimated to occur in five cases per 10 000 discectomies, i.e. it is very rare.

4   Mortality figures are:

- Aortic perforation: 78%.
- Inferior vena cava perforation: 89%.
- Iliac vessel perforation offers a slightly better survival, i.e. it is catastrophic.

5   Management of this problem. Clearly fluid resuscitation with large-bore intravenous lines is essential and should commence immediately. Cross-matched blood should be ordered straight away. Get another anaesthetist to help, especially if invasive monitoring is at all feasible. However, once the diagnosis of a tear in a major vessel is made then a laparotomy, with control of the haemorrhage by clamping of the vessel, is required urgently, otherwise the patient may not survive. There is no place for any imaging to confirm the diagnosis. You may be faced with difficult choices if a vascular surgeon is not immediately available and consideration should be given to a non-specialist opening the abdomen to clamp the vessel while waiting for the vascular surgeon.

Scenario 6

1   Immediate management. An inadvertent dural tap has obviously occurred. Three main options are available for analgesia:

- Abandoning further attempts at regional analgesia.
- Removing the Tuohy needle and attempting to resite an epidural at another space.
- Passing an epidural catheter through the existing needle and thereafter providing continuous subarachnoid analgesia with intermittent boluses of local ± opioid.

As soon as is practicable after the occurrence of the dural tap, a full and frank explanation should be offered to the patient. Consideration should be given at this time to the patient's state of mind. The explanation may have to be repeated once the patient is comfortable and able to assimilate the information given to her. Whenever possible she should be involved in deciding which of the above options are taken. Few anaesthetists would choose to abandon a regional technique unless it was thought that subsequent attempts to resite an epidural would prove impossible or were likely to result in a further dural puncture. Resiting the epidural at another interspace (usually at a higher space) is probably the most commonly used option at present. Care should be taken with subsequent top-ups as unpredictably high spread may occur. For this reason many units advocate the use of reduced-dose top-ups given by the anaesthetist (rather than the midwife) with careful monitoring of block height. Increasingly common is the use of intermittent subarachnoid boluses of low-dose local anaesthetic often with a small dose of opioid. The anaesthetist obviously should administer these with care, as above. This technique has the potential advantage of decreasing the incidence of post-dural puncture headache (PDPH), although this is controversial. It was previously common practice to subsequently deliver the child with forceps, or to place a limit on the time allowed for maternal expulsive efforts. This was thought to decrease the subsequent incidence of headache. This practice has virtually been abandoned and labour should be allowed to progress as previously planned. Some authorities recommend epidural infusion of saline post delivery in an attempt to decrease the incidence of headache.

2 This patient is obviously at risk of developing a PDPH. The incidence in this patient population with a needle of this size is in excess of 70%. Treatment of PDPH is initially symptomatic. The patient should be reassured and the earlier explanation reiterated. Maintenance of hydration, simple analgesics and caffeine is the mainstay of early treatment. Prophylactic bed rest is no longer recommended, but it may provide temporary symptomatic relief. If headache is still troublesome after 24 hours, epidural blood patch is the treatment of choice. This is effective in 90% of cases after one patch and 95% after a second. If there are any contraindications to this, bearing in mind the patient may be reluctant to undergo a further attempt at epidural space location, infusion of saline into the epidural space is an alternative that may be tried.

3 Although not used, an alternative solution would have been to initially perform a subarachnoid block using an atraumatic needle with a low-dose, local anaesthetic/opioid mixture. Once this block was established it would have allowed better patient cooperation, decreasing the likelihood of the patient moving unpredictably. However, this still involves breaching the dura, with the subsequent risks (albeit comparatively reduced) of unpredictable spread and, indeed, headache.

Further reading

Duffy PJ, Crosby ET. The epidural blood patch: resolving the controversies. *Can J Anaesth* 1999; 46(9): 878–886

Sajjad T, Ryan TD. Current management of inadvertent dural taps occurring during the siting of epidurals for pain relief in labour: a survey of maternity units in the United Kingdom. *Anaesthesia* 1995; 50(2): 156–161

1 Anaesthetic management: Options for control of the airway are:

- Awake fibre-optic intubation.
- Intubation under deep gaseous anaesthesia.
- Tracheostomy under local anaesthesia.

A full assessment of the airway is made. Experienced help should be sought and blood should be grouped and saved.

If awake, fibre-optic intubation is planned; a careful preoperative explanation of the procedure should be given. Sedative premedication is avoided. An antisialogogue may reduce swallowing and increase the effectiveness of topical anaesthetics. After establishing intravenous access and monitoring, the nasal mucosa is anaesthetized with ribbon soaked in cocaine. The oral cavity may be anaesthetized by gargling with 4% lignocaine. A cricothyroid injection of local anaesthetic may be performed if the area is free of tumour. The bronchoscope is introduced through the nose with a small internal diameter endotracheal tube railroaded over it. Care is taken to avoid bleeding. Further local anaesthetic may be sprayed if required as the bronchoscope is advanced through the nasopharynx, oropharynx and vocal cords and into the trachea. Position is confirmed by a view of the carina. After the airway is secured, the patient may be anaesthetized with an intravenous agent.

Gaseous induction may be attempted using halothane or sevoflurane in oxygen; the procedure must be abandoned if the airway becomes obstructed as anaesthesia deepens. The surgeon performing the tracheostomy should be on standby if the airway becomes acutely compromised during the procedure. If laryngoscopy proves impossible, a blind nasal intubation may rarely be successful.

Tracheostomy may be performed under local anaesthesia as a third option or should the above options fail.

Many surgeons would perform the gastrostomy before the tracheostomy formation. Anaesthesia can be maintained with volatile agent, short-acting opioid and medium-acting muscle relaxant, although intravenous techniques are acceptable alternatives. There may be technical difficulty inserting the endoscope into the oesophagus for PEG formation owing to tumour infiltration, but otherwise the PEG is usually unchallenging for the patient. The head is fully extended for the tracheostomy. After dissection down to the trachea the patient is pre-oxygenated and the oral cavity suctioned. If the insertion is likely to be prolonged, an intravenous anaesthetic technique will become necessary. The endotracheal tube is withdrawn under the direct vision of the surgeon, so that the tip is still below the cords; the tracheostomy tube is then inserted and its correct position may be confirmed with the bronchoscope prior to ventilation through it. Postoperatively the patient is nursed semi-recumbent and humidified oxygen is administered. A chest X-ray is done to confirm correct positioning of the tracheostomy tube and to exclude a pneumothorax. The tube is secured firmly and a tracheal dilator is made immediately available.

2   The complications of tracheostomy are as follows:
    Early:

- Bleeding (superficial or deep).
- Hypoxia.
- Surgical emphysema.
- Pneumothorax.
- Pneumomediastinum.
- Malposition of the tube.
- Tube obstruction.
- Laryngeal nerve damage.
- Tracheal tear.
- Mucosal flap.

Intermediate:

- Tube obstruction or displacement.
- Secondary haemorrhage.
- Infection.

Late:

- Infection.
- Obstruction.
- Erosion into cartilage, major vessel or oesophagus.
- Subglottic stenosis.
- Scar formation.

Further reading

Crosby ET, Cooper RM, Douglas MT et al. The unanticipated difficult airway with recommendations for management. *Can J Anaesth* 1998; 45(8): 757–776

Scenario 8

1   Muscle weakness may have been precipitated by the recent efforts of labour and subsequent increased workload involved in caring for a newborn baby. This would be a myasthenic crisis. In this case labour was uneventful and not prolonged. Azathioprine may be reduced in pregnancy, resulting in precipitation of symptoms. This would again be a myasthenic crisis. In this case the usual dose of azathioprine was maintained. Although there was no history of postnatal depression or overdose, this possibility cannot be ruled out. Overdose of pyridostigmine would produce a cholinergic crisis. An underlying infection, aminoglycoside therapy or magnesium sulphate enemas can all provoke severe weakness.

2   The patient requires urgent ventilatory support for respiratory distress. A rapid-sequence induction is appropriate – swallowing may be impaired if there is bulbar muscle weakness. Thiopentone and suxamethonium (see below) are suitable agents. The patient may require resuscitation with intravenous fluids prior to induction – dehydration may be present if swallowing has been impaired for a prolonged period. The patient requires ventilatory support on the intensive care unit. No further relaxant is given.

3   Preoperative assessment is aimed at assessing swallowing (if there is bulbar involvement) and the ability to cough and clear secretions. Preoperative investigations include chest X-ray (to exclude aspiration, infection or thymoma), arterial blood gases and respiratory function tests. Bulbar and respiratory weakness may indicate a need for postoperative ventilation. Always consider whether a regional technique is feasible.

Premedication with atropine may be used to reduce secretions: steroid cover may be required. Anticholinesterase treatment should be reduced on the day of surgery.

Anaesthesia is induced with a small dose of intravenous induction agent. The response of the neuromuscular junction is determined prior to giving relaxants. Intubation may be achieved under deep volatile anaesthesia: one dose of suxamethonium may be used. There is usually a normal response to depolarizing relaxants but fasciculations may not occur. Myasthenics are very sensitive to non-depolarizing muscle relaxants, resulting in prolonged action and incomplete reversal. Non-depolarizing relaxants are avoided – if this is not possible, from one-tenth to one-quarter of the normal dose of atracurium is the relaxant of choice, allowing return of neuromuscular function without active reversal. Quinine, aminoglycosides, ciprofloxacin and hypokalaemia all potentiate myasthenia and should be avoided.

If thymectomy is being performed, there is risk of pneumothorax and trauma to the superior vena cava – a large-bore pedal cannula is sited before the start of surgery.

Postoperatively, elective ventilation is advisable for 24–48 hours after major surgery, with regular chest physiotherapy and tracheal suction. Anticholinesterase treatment is restarted – the initial dose needed may be less than preoperatively.

These patients may be immunosuppressed as a result of medical therapy.

Further reading

Baraka A, Siddik S, Kawkabani N. Cisatracurium in a myasthenic patient undergoing thymectomy. *Can J Anaesth* 1999; 46(8): 779–782

Lorimer M, Hall R. Remifentanil and propofol total intravenous anaesthesia for thymectomy in myasthenia gravis. *Anaesth Intensive Care* 1998; 26(2): 210–212

Naguib M, el Dawlatly AA, Ashour M, Bamgboye EA. Multivariate determinants of the need for postoperative ventilation in myasthenia gravis. *Can J Anaesth* 1996; 43(10): 1006–1013

Nates JL, Cooper DJ, Day B, Tuxen DV. Acute weakness syndromes in critically ill patients—a reappraisal. *Anaesth Intensive Care* 1997; 25(5): 502–513

Scenario 9

1   The likely cause is choanal atresia. This may be complete of partial, unilateral or bilateral, but because the neonate is an obligate nasal breather, when the mouth is closed apnoea occurs. The passage of a soft suction catheter

through both sides of the nose is attempted. Failure to pass into the oropharyngx is highly suggestive.

2 Preservation of an oral airway is essential. The use of oral airways is most commonly effective, but endotracheal intubation may be necessary. An urgent paediatric ENT opinion is needed.

3 The olfactory pit is formed between the medial and lateral nasal swellings. The formation of the primary palate is associated with rupture of the bucconasal membranes to form the primitive choanae. Following this rupture the maxillary palatal folds develop and ultimately fuse to form the secondary palate. Migration of mesoderm into this area forms the bony and soft tissues of the nasal septum and the sphenoid pterygoid bones. Failure of rupture of the bucconasal membrane may result in partial or complete failure or normal posterior nasal development.

4 This condition is occasionally associated with cardiac abnormalities. These may be both structural and related to the conductive system. Cardiological assessment using echocardiography and a 12-lead ECG is essential, and should precede surgery. There is a rare possibility of tracheomalacia in these neonates, but this will not be seen until the nasal obstruction has been treated.

5 The surgical treatment depends on whether this is complete or partial atresia. If complete, the surgeon will try to fracture the anterolateral border of the sphenoid bone – the pterygoid hamulus area – and open a direct route into the oropharynx. If there is only partial atresia he will dilate the nasal airway with bougies. This often fractures the vomer, first to one side and then to the other, and is not believed to be as effective as fracturing the more robust sphenoid pterygoid bones. The nasal airway is then preserved with nasal stents – usually a cut endotracheal tube.

6 Anaesthetic management is based on the need to preserve the oral airway during induction. Full monitoring prior to induction is mandatory to elucidate any conduction problems or bradycardia that develops. Atropine 20 μg kg^{-1} should be administered preoperatively, and a gaseous induction is the commonest method chosen. Once the neonate is stable, intravenous access is gained. The procedure is seldom short, and endotracheal intubation and protection of the lower airway by packing is advised. The postoperative period is often safe, but the unstable control of breathing at this age makes monitoring with apnoea monitors and pulse oximetry wise.

After 3–6 weeks the surgeon will want to remove the stents and perform an EUA of the posterior nasal space. Anaesthesia for removal of the stents may be hazardous, as they may prevent effective sealing of the mask and reduce the efficiency of manual assisted ventilation. There is still a risk of airway contamination and endotracheal intubation is necessary. The airway may be initially worse than preoperatively and paediatric high-dependency unit or ICU care is recommended.

Scenario 10

1 The likeliest diagnosis is obstructive sleep apnoea syndrome (OSA).

2 BMI is weight (in kilograms), divided by the square of his height (in metres).

3   These patients are unable to maintain their airway when asleep or when anaesthetized. They usually have decreased reflex responses to hypoxia and hypercarbia, and are extremely sensitive to sedative or opiate premedication (to the point of respiratory arrest). They may have right ventricular failure because of the profound pulmonary hypertension the episodes of arterial oxygen desaturation cause. They are often grossly obese and this compounds the effects of their fragile control of their airway.

Induction of anaesthesia will be immediately followed by the loss of airway patency, rapid desaturation and severe pulmonary hypertension. The predisposing factors to sleep apnoea are similar to those associated with a predicted difficult intubation – large tongue, recessive jaw, long palate, for example. Their poor ventilatory drive and almost absent chemical reflex control predispose them to profound hypoventilation during anaesthesia.

They remain unable to maintain their airway until fully awake, and are particularly at risk in the early postoperative period – in the recovery ward. They are most vulnerable during REM sleep stages, and will remain at an increased risk until the delayed REM rebound that occurs following surgery has resolved. This is usually after the third postoperative night.

4   Cancel the patient's operation. Arrange to borrow a pulse oximeter from theatre, and measure his saturation overnight. (The majority of oximeters have a memory, and this can be printed out in the morning.) The recording will be very useful in confirming the diagnosis. The patient needs urgent referral to you nearest sleep investigations unit. Inform both the surgeon and the patient's GP of your concerns. The GP may need to consider the safety of this patient driving, for instance.

5   The sleep laboratory will perform overnight sleep studies. These will include pulse oximetry, ECG, a measure of breathing such as induction plethysmography, air flow, sound, video surveillance and sleep staging (this requires EEG, EOG and EMG signals). The diagnosis is made from observing the pattern of obstructive breathing patterns, severe oxyhaemoglobin desaturations and frequent arousals on the sleep staging. Sleep questionnaires are often also used to try to quantitate sleepiness, and to demonstrate effective treatment.

5   If the diagnosis is confirmed, the most effective treatment is nasal continuous positive airway pressure (CPAP). This treatment must be used every night, and for life. The effect of weight loss is usually great but takes far too long to be an immediate and safe alternative. The nasal CPAP must be used for at least 2 weeks before any elective surgery, and ideally for a month. The patient should bring his system with him to the theatre for use in the recovery unit, as well as in the surgical ward.

Further reading

Benumof JL. Obstructive sleep apnoea in the adult obese patient: implications for airway management. *J Clin Anaesth* 2001; 103(2): 144–156

Loadsman JA, Hillman DR. Anaesthesia and sleep apnoea. *Br J Anaesth* 2001; 86(2): 254–266

Index

Index

Index

Index

Index

Index

Index

Index

Index

Index